Sustainable Sexual Health

This book provides a textual analysis of the implementation of the UN's Sustainable Development Goals (SDGs) in health care.

Using sexual health as a case study, the authors apply Foucault's notions of biopower and biopolitics to discuss the power struggle between local needs and wants and universal ambitions embedded in the SDG ideology. Reproductive and sexual health are settings where health policy, religious and cultural norms, and gender policy meet personal and moral standards. As such, tensions, dilemmas, and conflicts are powerfully demonstrated in this interdisciplinary field of public health. Tensions, dilemmas, and conflicts are particularly visible in reproductive and sexual health settings, where health policy meets personal or moral standards, gender policy, and religious and cultural norms.

This book will be valuable supplementary material for graduate students and academics wishing to enhance their knowledge in the fields of global health, sexual health, reproductive health and rights, and cultural studies. The book will also be of interest to professionals and students within the disciplines of medical sociology, medical anthropology, sustainability studies, gender and sexuality studies, and public health.

Tony Sandset is a research fellow at the Centre for Sustainable Healthcare Education (SHE) at the Faculty of Medicine, University of Oslo, where he received his PhD in cultural history. His current research focuses on knowledge translation within the field of HIV care and prevention. Specifically, his focus is on how medical knowledge from randomized controlled trials is mediated, how evidence is generated in HIV prevention, and how new medical technologies inform subjectivities, desire, and sexuality. Another of his research areas pertains to the intersection between race, gender, class, and HIV care and prevention. Relating race, class, and gender to how medical knowledge is disseminated and translated from research to clinical and community usage is of particular interest here.

Eivind Engebretsen is a full professor of interdisciplinary health science (with emphasis on the philosophy of science) at the University of Oslo (UoO). He is currently the Vice-Dean for Postgraduate Studies at the Faculty of Medicine. In his research, Engebretsen has pioneered new approaches to the study of the interfaces of political ideologies (including SDGs) and knowledge production in health care, drawing on political philosophy and discourse analysis. His work has been awarded with a fellowship from the Centre for Advanced Study at the Norwegian Academy of Science and Letters. He is Founding Chair of the Faculty of Medicine's Centre of Excellence in Sustainable Healthcare Education.

Kristin Heggen is a professor in health sciences, University of Oslo. From 2011–2018, she served as Dean of Education at the Faculty of Medicine, University of Oslo. Heggen has expertise in the humanities, social sciences, and educational research. Her research interests include ethical issues and power dynamics, issues concerning knowledge production in health care, knowledge transfer between academic and clinical settings, and education of health professionals. She is currently Director of the Faculty of Medicine's Centre of Excellence in Sustainable Healthcare Education.

Routledge Studies in Public Health

Available titles include:

Conceptualising Public Health
Historical and Contemporary Struggles over Key Concepts
Edited by Johannes Kananen, Sophy Bergenheim, Merle Wessel

Global Health and Security
Critical Feminist Perspectives
Edited by Colleen O'Manique and Pieter Fourie

Women's Health and Complementary and Integrative Medicine
Edited by Jon Adams, Amie Steel, Alex Broom and Jane Frawley

Managing the Global Health Response to Epidemics
Social Science Perspectives
Edited by Mathilde Bourrier, Nathalie Brender and Claudine Burton-Jeangros

The Anthropology of Tobacco
Ethnographic Adventures in Non-Human Worlds
Edited by Mathilde Bourrier, Nathalie Brender and Claudine Burton-Jeangros

Public Health Evaluation and the Social Determinants of Health
Kelley Allyson

Sustainable Sexual Health
Analysing the Implementation of the SDGs
Tony Sandset, Eivind Engebretsen and Kristin Heggen

Dementia in Prison
An Ethical Framework to Support Research, Practice and Prisoners
Joanne Brooke

www.routledge.com/Routledge-Studies-in-Public-Health/book-series/RSPH

Sustainable Sexual Health

Analysing the Implementation of the SDGs

Tony Sandset, Eivind Engebretsen and Kristin Heggen

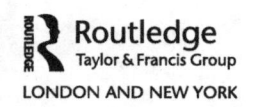

LONDON AND NEW YORK

First published 2021
by Routledge
2 Park Square, Milton Park, Abingdon, Oxon OX14 4RN

and by Routledge
52 Vanderbilt Avenue, New York, NY 10017

Routledge is an imprint of the Taylor & Francis Group, an informa business

British Library Cataloguing-in-Publication Data
A catalogue record for this book is available from the British Library

Library of Congress Cataloging-in-Publication Data
A catalog record for this book has been requested

ISBN: 978-0-367-17907-6 (hbk)
ISBN: 978-0-429-05621-5 (ebk)

Typeset in Times New Roman
by Apex CoVantage, LLC

Contents

Acknowledgments

Although the authors take full responsibility for this manuscript, the book itself benefited from the efforts of many inspiring and engaged colleagues who deserve public credit.

Important members of our multidisciplinary research group Knowledge in Translation (KNOWIT) have been involved in numerous discussions related to the core ideas of our project. This research group is affiliated with the Faculty of Medicine at the University of Oslo in Norway and focuses on knowledge translation in health policy and health care practices. Our book focuses on the tensions, dilemmas, and conflicts which are typically contested in sexual health, an area where policy and evidence meet personal and moral standards. Members of KNOWIT have contributed with enthusiasm for a long time to our project in major ways – as resource persons for our research topics, theoretical and analytical approaches, and – probably most importantly – as critical friends. We want to express special thanks to Ida Lillehagen, Gina Fraas Henrichsen, Sietse Wieringa, Clemet Askheim, Carolina Borges Rau Steuernagel, Hilde Ousland Vandeskog, and John Ødemark.

During the last couple of years, we have, as a group, been complemented by several other researchers from University of Oslo, as well as international universities. We would, as such, extend our thanks to Professor Trisha Greenhalgh at Oxford University for her continual support and inspirational ideas. In Sweden, at the Karolinska Institute, we have enjoyed the inspirational and intellectual support of Professor Göran Tomson and Professor Ole Petter Ottesen.

A common focus for all of us has been our interests in and focus on the implementation of the United Nations' Sustainable Development Goals (SDGs). An interest of ours has thus been various challenges to knowledge translation, including tensions between local and global concerns, as well as potential conflicts between social and economic dimensions of health. A grant application for a center of excellence in education was crowned with success in 2019, and the Centre for Sustainable Healthcare Education (SHE) became a reality. For the next ten years, the center will offer several opportunities to further develop the research presented in this book and include these important knowledge areas in future education of health professionals.

We would also like to extend our gratitude to the editors at Routledge and to Evie Lonsdale for all her continual support along the way in taking this book from manuscript form to a book.

Finally, yet importantly, we would like to express our gratitude to the Centre for Advanced Study (CAS) at the Norwegian Academy of Science and Letters. We have been fortunate to spend the autumn of 2019 and the spring semester 2020 at this center, which is an independent foundation that furthers excellent, fundamental, curiosity-driven research. We have truly enjoyed the hospitality and support offered by the center, which has been invaluable in offering the time to finish the manuscript for this book.

1 Introduction

Background and contexts: sustainability as carnal policies

The main outcome of the UN 2030 Agenda was the development of seventeen Sustainable Development Goals (SDGs) which aim to secure health and well-being for all humans (United Nations, 2015). The SDGs were adopted by all 193 member states of the UN in 2015 and will lead to a unique mobilization of human and financial resources towards an ambitious "plan of action for people, planet and prosperity." Governments, the public and private sectors, and non-governmental organizations (NGOs) are expected to form a "collaborative partnership" in order to realize the plan, which pledges that "no one will be left behind." Of the seventeen goals, one, goal three, is specifically dedicated to health, while several others explicitly address the environmental, political, social, and economic determinants of health and well-being. The SDGs thus represent a paradigm shift from the relatively selective focus on specific diseases found in the Millennium Development Goals (MDGs) towards a holistic vision of health and well-being (Buse & Hawkes, 2015; United Nations, 2015).

The push towards reaching the 2030 SDGs has been spearheaded by a consensus-driven agenda that all member states have agreed to follow and implement within their respective localized national contexts. The journey from a global agenda to local implementation can, however, lead to conflicts between different actors. Global principles and values sometimes clash with localized needs, values, and concerns; evidence-based policies strive for hegemony over local, tacit, and communal regimes of knowledge; and individual needs and desires compete with national and international ideas about what is best for the individual in the name of sustainable health and sustainability writ large. Tensions, dilemmas, and conflicts are especially contested in reproductive and sexual health, where health policy meets personal and moral standards and brings in gender concerns, as well as family concerns and religious and cultural norms in tension with official policies.

This book will focus on the ways in which sexual health, in the era of the SDGs, has become an important term within global health. In doing so, we also want to shed light on some of the power struggles that exist between local needs and wants and the universal ambitions embedded in the ideology of the SDGs. The book will also focus on the productive role that *texts and documents* have in the implementation process of sexual health policies and the SDGs. Implementation of the SDGs and sexual health policies is dependent on texts in various formats on different levels. Ranging from UN policy documents to national, regional, and local implementation plans, guidelines, and implementation reports, the place of textual documents in the implementation of both the SDGs and sexual health strategies should not be underestimated.

We have chosen to work with case studies, which rather than mere examples represent places or areas of reflection where the SDGs have come to influence issues ranging from HIV/AIDS prevention to reproductive health, as well as broader notions of human sexuality and its connection to health. As such, the chapters in this book should not be read as a linear model for conceptualizing how the SDGs have come to influence the idea of sexual health, nor should the book be seen as offering an exhaustive and final overview of the topic at hand. Rather, the book offers an illuminating site for exploration of how sustainable development and sexual health relate. Hence, the chapters to come can be read as standalone case studies analyzing the specific topics at hand rather than simple reflections of the broader narrative of sustainable development and sexual health. We think that this offers a better way of discerning the nuances and effects that are played out when the concept of sustainable development meets with, and is combined with, sexual health. To underline the importance of our chosen case studies, we should also make clear at the outset that the rise and proliferation of the concept of sexual health have become a focal point in many international and national strategic plans concerned with public health and sustainability. Sexual health has come to occupy a privileged position within public health domains. From local clinics and public pedagogy in schools to the World Health Organization (WHO) and the UN, sexual health has engendered ways to intervene in, discipline, and regulate not only health but also sexual behavior, including efforts and advice aimed at disciplining individuals to act in responsible ways and following recommendations for sustainable health. Sexual health thus represents a concept that has important consequences for how the state and the subject must stand in relationship to each other.

As such, sexual health as an object of knowledge, policy, and public concern rests on this important tension between the state on the one hand and the individual on the other. This is why we contend that sexual health has become an object of inquiry and importance within the SDG discourses; there cannot be a sustainable future at the global level if the very localized level of personal intimacy and health is also not made sustainable. Hence, we see a strong incongruity between the grand and global ambitions of the SDGs on the one hand and, on the other hand, the localized and very personal intimacy found in sexual and reproductive health. In other words, in terms of the sustainability equation, there is a tension between the universal and global on one side and the local, personal, and minute intimacy of the subject on the other. We maintain that the concept of sexual health also includes reproductive health. This is in line with the new synchronized definition offered by the WHO (WHO, 2002, 2016). With this position, this book also takes seriously the SDG agenda's premise that an increased focus on and effort to facilitate access to sexual and reproductive health services are prerequisites to the implementation of the SDG goals (e.g. targets 3.7 and 5.7). These targets are also operationalized in a recent WHO white paper (WHO, 2016). It is a paradox that to reach the UN's grand and all-encompassing promise to "leave no one behind" when it comes to global sustainable (sexual) health, we must turn to the most private of moments, in which these interventions finally must reside. It is in the moment of sexual intimacy between two individuals that global sustainability finally is acted out. Put differently, if the UN is to fulfill its global promise of sustainable sexual health, these grand implementation strategies must inevitably target the most private of spaces; thus, there is an interesting juxtaposition between the grand scope and ambitions of the SDGs and their final target, namely the micro-space of human intimacy.[1]

As part of the SDGs, sexual health can be seen as the site at which life meets death. Sex – specifically the moment of sexual intercourse – has the potential to bring new vitality into the world through reproduction and children, which represent a possible sustainable future. However, this moment also represents the antithesis of sustainability, namely entropy and death. This is most clear in the case of HIV/AIDS infections as a harbinger of death and morbidity, but reproduction also becomes a space wherein death is a potential outcome. Finally, reproduction can be a source of concern due to the haunting ghost of overpopulation, a concern that is a potential problem for the entire globe and not just the person or family.

Power and politics in global health: a backdrop for the Sustainable Development Goals and sexual health

Many scholars have highlighted the role of politics and power in global health. This includes forms of power that are widespread but little analyzed and debated, such as power perceived as legitimate "by virtue of [its] grounding in knowledge or humanitarian motives" (Shiffman, 2014, pp. 32–36). Even so-called humanitarian interventions can be read as being carried out both through an idea of care and a language based on threats (Feldman & Ticktin, 2010). Thus, even within the discourse of sustainability, and in particular when interventions are made in the name of sustainability, we maintain that power and authority are key issues that need to be addressed and looked at critically. In particular, the power to make decisions about one's own body and health becomes key in an age when there is more and more reliance on evidence-based medicine and best-practice policies, many of which rest on neo-liberal philosophical underpinnings. Researchers have argued that liberal forms of power have become increasingly important in global health governance (Engebretsen & Heggen, 2014). In keeping with this claim, research has also pointed to an "audit explosion," and the systems of self-regulation that this explosion has engendered have created new and indirect forms of governance (Power, 1997). As Nikolas Rose has articulated so well, governance has, to a large extent, become governance of self-governance (Rose, 1999). This is relevant to the field of health policy analysis, as well as to implementation studies which see the relationship between the state and the individual as hinging on a certain form of governmentality (Foucault, 2007, 2008) wherein health care advice, health promotions, and general public health efforts are increasingly based on the dissemination of health information through media channels, infomercials, and public health promotions (Armstrong, 1995; Race, 2008; Karlsen & Villadsen, 2016). This is a form of power which operates not only through knowledge and norms but also, and often unconsciously, through language and concepts (Stone, 1997; Engebretsen & Heggen, 2015), which, as we will argue throughout this book, are highly relevant ways of thinking through how power works within the implementation of the SDGs and their health targets found in the discourse on sexual health.

A related criticism concerns the use of and reliance on metrics in global health politics. Critics have claimed that indicators do not just measure results but also govern activities, which end up being adapted to whatever results can be measured (Power, 1997; Foucault, 2007; Porter, 2013; Adams, 2016; Davis, 2017; Fukuda-Parr & Yamin, 2017). This has been the basis of certain criticisms directed at the predecessors of the SDGs, the MDGs, and their alleged success (Adams, 2016; Roalkvam & McNeill, 2016). Scholars have claimed that improving scores become more important than improving people's lives (Pogge, 2013; Weber, 2015; Hickel, 2016; Davis, 2017), a criticism that is still highly relevant in connection with the SDGs and their work on, for instance, reducing the rate of new HIV infections. An emblematic example here would be the case of UNAIDS, which still uses the saying "what gets measured gets done."[2]

Other relevant criticisms of the SDGs have been made by authors who have commented on the lack of public engagement or campaigning for the SDGs and the lack of political activism related to the Agenda (Labonté, 2016; Ruckert et al., 2017; Saiz & Donald, 2017; van de Pas, 2017). Still others have pointed to the importance of a vibrant and engaged civil society (Smith et al., 2016; Williams & Taylor, 2017). Some researchers are also concerned with power, ideology, and politics related to the SDGs (Weber, 2014; Labonté, 2016; Scheyvens et al., 2016). Weber, for instance, examined the extent to which the ambition expressed in the Agenda to "leave no one behind" is premised on neoliberalism (Weber, 2017). While we also stand by this criticism to a certain extent in the following, we will also move beyond it, turning our analytical gaze to emerging paradoxes and tensions rather than firmly entrenching our conversation within a critique of the SDGs as neoliberal handmaidens.

Another key insight would be the formulation of an analytical framework that can account for the ambiguities that are embedded within the very term "sustainability." Engebretsen et al. have drawn attention to some of the ambiguities inherent in both the SDGs and the concept of sustainability and emphasized that these ambiguities can complicate the implementation process by glossing over divergent ideological positions (Engebretsen et al., 2016, 2017). The risk of neglecting certain groups of the world's population is also discussed and will be highlighted in this book, in particular when dealing with HIV/AIDS and its role concerning the SDGs and sustainability. Thus, these issues of power and inequality and the clash between local norms, values, beliefs, and needs and alleged universal, rational, and global knowledge and desires in terms of what can be considered sustainable will be of key interest in the chapters to come.

Theoretical influence

Our theoretical influence comes primarily from Michel Foucault and his concepts of biopower and biopolitics. Foucault first introduced biopower as an analytical concept during his lectures at the Collège de France in the late 1970s (Foucault, 2003, 2007, 2008). The concept also appears in his work on the history of sexuality, in particular volume one of that series (Foucault, 1998). For Foucault, biopower began with a change in how power operates within Western European countries in the 17th century:

> I think that one of the greatest transformations political right underwent in the nineteenth century was precisely that, I wouldn't say exactly sovereignty's old right – to take life or let live – was replaced, but it came to be complemented by a new right which does not erase the old right but which does penetrate it, permeate it. This is the right, or rather precisely the opposite right. It is the power to "make" live and "let" die. The right of sovereignty was the right to take life or let live. And then this new right is established: the right to make live and to let die.
>
> (Foucault, 2003, p. 241)

No longer was the sovereign power of the state that of being able to decide who was to die and who was to live; rather, that power was now extended to influence and decide who should live, what kind of life they were to live, and under what circumstances these lives were to be able to prosper and develop. In short, biopower describes the moment in time when politics became enmeshed with "life" in all its forms and functions. The effects of the process through which these mutations in the exercise of power occurred can be characterized as having formed two opposite poles of a continuum. The first of these occurred through the development of techniques that operated in and on the individual body: "that discipline tries to rule a multiplicity of men to the extent that their multiplicity can and must be dissolved into individual bodies that can be kept under surveillance, trained, used, and . . . punished" (Foucault, 2003, p. 242). This pole is referred to as "anatamo-politics," and it is chiefly concerned with the atomization of a collectivity for governance and productivity to a certain end. The second pole is of explicitly biopolitics, concerning the whole of a population, with the ultimate effect being characterizable as "massifying, that is directed not at man-as-body but as man-as-species" (Foucault, 2003, p. 243). Even though biopower's techniques of power are concentrated at the level of national, and even global, populations, it needs another pole, which is that of a set of disciplining techniques aimed at the body of the individual. Here the techniques are aimed at producing individualizing effects and manipulating the body in such a way that it is a resource and at the same time becomes docile (Foucault in Campbell &

Sitze, 2013, p. 69). Foucault mentions disciplining techniques used in schools, the military, and factories as key (Foucault, 2012); however, the health advice that emerges from instruction on hygiene and public advice on sexuality and fertility is but one of the techniques that also inscribe themselves on the body of the subject (Foucault, 2008). Thus, biopower centers on the subject but employs two poles to produce, or at least try to produce, a productive yet docile body: one is disciplinary, and the other is regulatory; one is preoccupied with the individual, and the other takes the population as its main target.

In following Foucault and his take on biopower, we contend that policies that aim to promote "sustainable sexual health" can usefully be analyzed as biopolitics par excellence insofar as the policy documents that we have analyzed implicitly state that for the State to survive and become sustainable, its population needs to adopt sustainable sexual health habits. But this is because these documents form a powerful strategy that follows the two poles of Foucault's biopower; they are at once disciplinary, targeting bodies and subjects, and regulatory at the level of the body politic, targeting the population as a whole.

We contend that these documents employ both a regulatory and normalizing approach to sexual and reproductive health and an approach that is meant to discipline the subject. They do so by following a particular logic of evidence-based knowledge that we contend can be detrimental to the empowering underpinnings of the UN's SDGs in that it produces not a plethora of voices but rather a narrow set of guidelines that subjects are to follow when it comes to cultivating sustainable sexual health for themselves and, by extension, the State.

However, we cannot avoid a second reason for choosing to work with Foucault's concepts of biopower and biopolitics, which is the connection Foucault himself makes between sex and biopower. As Foucault notes, sex is key in how it allows for biopolitical interventions at both the individual level and at the population level; it fuses the disciplinary power which targets the individual body and the regulatory power aimed at the population level:

> This is the background that enables us to understand the importance assumed by sex as a political issue. It was at the pivot of the two axes along which developed the entire political technology of life. On the one hand, it was tied to the disciplines of the body: the harnessing, intensification, and distribution of forces, the adjustment, and economy of energies. On the other hand, it was applied to the regulation of populations, through all the far-reaching effects of its activity. It fitted in both categories at once, giving rise to infinitesimal surveillances, permanent controls, extremely meticulous orderings of space, indeterminate medical or psychological examinations, to an entire micropower concerned with the body. But it gave rise as well to comprehensive measures, statistical assessments, and interventions aimed at the entire social body or groups taken as a whole. Sex was a means of access both to the life of the body and the life of the species. It was employed as a standard for the disciplines and as a basis for regulations.
>
> (Foucault, 1990, pp. 145–146)

In light of this, we also contend that the new focus on sexual health, in combination with a focus on sustainability and ideology of evidence-based policy, logically would target sex because sex allows for health policy interventions that target both the individual body in a disciplining manner and the population at a regulatory level. Sex, as the moment of reproduction, becomes, in the modern regime, a moment of explicit concern for the state, the future of which also depends on a steady, healthy, and continual supply of new citizens that are both productive and engaged with the state. In the SDGs, sex, as part of sexual and reproductive health, becomes a similar site of explicit concern, since it is the moment wherein both local or national concerns of vitality and entropy are played out and, indeed, the drama moves onto the global scene, where not only local or national biopolitical concerns are being formulated, but indeed global biopolitics are in play. This global biopolitics is under the auspices of either reaching a sustainable future for mankind or the very destruction of the foundation upon which our species rests, part of which is influenced by how we as subjects and as a species engage with sexuality and sex.

On the one hand, Foucault states that sexuality, being an eminently corporal form of behavior, is a matter of individualized disciplinary control that takes the form of continual self-surveillance which has been instilled through social norms in school, medical advice, and legal injunctions and other sources of sexual norms (Foucault, 2003, p. 251). On the other hand, because sexuality also carries population-based considerations, in particular through reproduction but also various diseases, it is also regulated through biopolitical techniques of power that target the population as well as the body of the individual (Foucault, 2003, p. 251). Here we contend that policy documents, national guidelines, and reports such as epidemiology and statistics are part and parcel of this biopower that targets sexual health at the individual level as well as at the population level. Foucault also notes that medicine, in particular, is a power-knowledge that, in connection to sexual health, can target both "the body and the population, the organism and the biological processes, and it will, therefore, have both disciplinary effects and regulatory effects" (Foucault, 2003, p. 252). Since we are concerned with how health policy documents intervene both in the lives of individuals and at the policy level of populations, our starting point in analyzing the documents that we have worked with will be as follows: sexual health policies that focus on sexual health as a matter of enhancement through evidence-based policies should not be applauded without looking critically at the modes in which they also produce what can be seen as disciplining and regulatory effects, which in turn can produce tensions between the subject and the state.

Thus, this book will hopefully contribute to a nuanced and critically informed reading of some of how the SDGs are implemented, and we hope that this novel and innovative theoretical framework will add to the critical conversations that are now gradually taking place looking at the SDGs as potentially antagonistic and paradoxical dicta that should not be taken at face value as just a series of benign interpellations of the people of the earth in the name of sustainability.

Concluding remarks

In sum, we are hopeful that these cases, in combination with our choice of framework, will illuminate new problematics that will allow the reader to take part in the critical discussion that is engendered by looking at the tensions and paradoxes that we try to show are unfolding within certain settings surrounding the construction of the SDGs. We also want to highlight the ideological and epistemological foundation upon which the SDGs themselves rest. Part of this is to highlight how sustainability has often come to mean quantification and metrics. We will try to highlight how this quantification, in turn, can be linked to a historical development wherein sustainability semantically has changed from a concept that in its early days focused on durability, while its later iterations have more and more come to mean the ability to self-improve and thus also imply a form of self-governance. Also, and perhaps too ambitiously, we hope that this book will contribute to an increase in both scholarship on and civic engagement with the SDGs, which in turn can lead to the development of a more democratic and power-sensitive approach to SDG implementation while at the same time providing an example of theoretical innovation and an exemplary case for the study and analysis of public health governance.

Notes

1 In the newer version of the concept of sexual health, reproductive health has come to be subsumed under and into the concept of sexual health. As such, the UN, the WHO, and others have at least signaled a more holistic definition of sexual health wherein the focus is no longer just on disease burden, mortality, and morbidity or dysfunction. Yet most reports that deal with these issues within the UN and WHO systems still focus on various diseases, child mortality rates, maternal death rates during pregnancy and delivery, and, to some degree, "sexual rights."
2 See the UNAIDS statement on data collection, the use of metrics, and the rationale for adhering to this dictum. www.unaids.org/en/topic/data

References

Adams, V. (2016). *Metrics: What counts in global health*. Duke University Press.
Armstrong, D. (1995). The rise of surveillance medicine. *Sociology of Health & Illness*, *17*(3), 393–404.
Bowen, A., & Casadevall, A. (2015). Increasing disparities between resource inputs and outcomes, as measured by certain health deliverables, in biomedical research. *Proceedings of the National Academy of Sciences*, *112*(36), 11335–11340.
Buse, K., & Hawkes, S. (2015). Health in the Sustainable Development Goals: Ready for a paradigm shift? *Globalization and Health*, *11*(13). https://doi.org/10.1186/s12992-015-0098-8.
Campbell, T., & Sitze, A. (2013). *Biopolitics: A reader*. Duke University Press.
Davis, S. L. (2017). The uncounted: Politics of data and visibility in global health. *The International Journal of Human Rights*, *21*(8), 1144–1163.
Engebretsen, E., & Heggen, K. (2014). Global governance for health: What about liberal power? *The Lancet*, *384*(9944), 664.

Engebretsen, E., & Heggen, K. (2015). Powerful concepts in global health: Comment on knowledge, moral claims, and the exercise of power in global health. *International Journal of Health Policy and Management, 4*(2), 115.

Engebretsen, E., Heggen, K., Das, S., Farmer, P., & Ottersen, O. P. (2016). Paradoxes of sustainability with consequences for health. *The Lancet Global Health, 4*(4), e225–e226.

Engebretsen, E., Heggen, K., & Ottersen, O. P. (2017). The Sustainable Development Goals: Ambiguities of accountability. *International Organization, 108,* 396–405.

Feldman, I., & Ticktin, M. (Eds.). (2010). *In the name of humanity: The government of threat and care.* Duke University Press.

Foucault, M. (1990). *The history of sexuality: An introduction.* Vintage.

Foucault, M. (1998). *The history of sexuality. Vol. 1: The will to knowledge.* Penguin Books.

Foucault, M. (2003). *"Society Must Be Defended": Lectures at the Collège de France, 1975–1976* (vol. 1). Macmillan.

Foucault, M. (2007). *Security, territory, population: Lectures at the Collège de France, 1977–78.* Springer.

Foucault, M. (2008). *The birth of biopolitics: Lectures at the Collège de France, 1978–1979.* Springer.

Foucault, M. (2012). *Discipline and punish: The birth of the prison.* Vintage.

Fukuda-Parr, S., & Yamin, A. E. (2017). *The MDGs, capabilities, and human rights: The power of numbers to shape agendas.* Routledge.

Hickel, J. (2016). The true extent of global poverty and hunger: Questioning the good news narrative of the millennium development goals. *Third World Quarterly, 37*(5), 749–767.

Karlsen, M. P., & Villadsen, K. (2016). Health promotion, governmentality, and the challenges of theorizing pleasure and desire. *Body & Society, 22*(3), 3–30.

Labonté, R. (2016). Health promotion in an age of normative equity and rampant inequality. *International Journal of Health Policy and Management, 5*(12), 675.

Pogge, T. (2013). Poverty, hunger, and cosmetic progress. In M. Langford, A. Sumner, & A. E. Yamin (Eds.), *The millennium development goals and human rights: Past, present, and future* (pp. 209–231). Cambridge University Press.

Porter, T. M. (2013). Funny numbers. *Culture Unbound: Journal of Current Cultural Research, 4*(4), 585–598.

Power, M. (1997). *The audit society: Rituals of verification.* Oxford University Press.

Race, K. (2008). The use of pleasure in harm reduction: Perspectives from the history of sexuality. *International Journal of Drug Policy, 19*(5), 417–423.

Roalkvam, S., & McNeill, D. (2016). What counts as progress? The contradictions of global health initiatives. *Forum for Development Studies, 43*(1), 68–88.

Rose, N. (1999). *Powers of freedom: Reframing political thought.* Cambridge University Press.

Ruckert, A., Schram, A., Labonté, R., Friel, S., Gleeson, D., & Thow, A. (2017). Policy coherence, health, and Sustainable Development Goals: A health impact assessment of the Trans-Pacific Partnership. *Critical Public Health, 27*(1), 86–96.

Saiz, I., & Donald, K. (2017). Tackling inequality through the Sustainable Development Goals: Human rights in practice. *The International Journal of Human Rights, 21*(8), 1029–1049.

Scheyvens, R., Banks, G., & Hughes, E. (2016). The private sector and the SDGs: The need to move beyond "business as usual". *Sustainable Development, 24*(6), 371–382.

Shiffman, J. (2014). Knowledge, moral claims, and the exercise of power in global health. *International Journal of Health Policy and Management, 3*(6), 297.

Smith, J., Buse, K., & Gordon, C. (2016). Civil society: The catalyst for ensuring health in the age of sustainable development. *Globalization and Health, 12*(1), 40. https://doi.org/10.1186/s12992-016-0178-4

Stone, D. A. (1997). *Policy paradox: The art of political decision making.* WW Norton.

United Nations. (2015). *Transforming our world: The 2030 agenda for sustainable development.* Resolution adopted by the General Assembly on 25: 70/1. Seventieth United Nations General Assembly.

van de Pas, R. (2017). Global health in the anthropocene: Moving beyond resilience and capitalism: Comment on health promotion in an age of normative equity and rampant inequality. *International Journal of Health Policy and Management, 6*(8), 481.

Weber, H. (2014). When goals collide: Politics of the MDGs and the post-2015 Sustainable Development Goals agenda. *SAIS Review of International Affairs, 34*(2), 129–139.

Weber, H. (2015). Reproducing inequalities through development: The MDGs and the politics of method. *Globalizations, 12*(4), 660–676.

Weber, H. (2017). Politics of "leaving no one behind": Contesting the 2030 Sustainable Development Goals agenda. *Globalizations, 14*(3), 399–414.

WHO. (2002). *Defining sexual health: Report of a technical consultation on sexual health.* WHO.

WHO. (2016). *Action plan for sexual and reproductive health: Towards achieving the 2030 agenda for sustainable development in Europe – leaving no one behind.* WHO.

Williams, B., & Taylor, S. (2017). Squaring the circle: Health as a bridge to global solidarity in the Sustainable Development Goals. *Archives of Disease in Childhood, 102*(5), 459–462.

2 The history, rise, and proliferation of "sustainability"

To more clearly understand the connection between the UN's Sustainable Development Goals and sexual health, a historical account of the two terms seems to be in order. We do this to chart out the historical emergence of both sustainability and sexual health to better understand why both of these concepts have become so prominent in public health. Second, and perhaps more importantly, we do this to show that the connection between the two concepts is an entangled history which has its starting point long before the SDGs came onto the scene in 2015. The current merger of sustainability and sexual health within the SDG framework is thus a new iteration of this entangled genealogy.

Sustainable development – a boundary concept of meaning

Sustainable development, as Grober states, sounds in many ways like the brainchild of a multinational commission, a formula achieved in the midnight hour of a tiring negotiation marathon (2007, p. 5). And, in many ways, sustainable development came onto the global stage in full force through the multinational UN in the aftermath of the 1992 Earth Summit in Rio de Janeiro and its Agenda 21 document (Grober, 2007, p. 5). The UN, in its Agenda 21 document, used the concept of sustainable development as a strategic concept meant to shape and save the "blue planet" as it heralded a new balance between the preservation of the potential of the natural world and its resources (Grober, 2007, p. 5; Grober & Cunningham, 2012). While the Earth Summit was key in launching sustainable development into the vocabulary of NGOs, national reports, and academic circles, as well as eventually becoming a concept that seemed to be on everyone's lips, its usage within the Agenda 21 document had already been foreshadowed in the by-now-famous Brundtland Commission, or, as it also was named, Our Common Future, from 1987. In it, the Brundtland Commission defined sustainable development as "development that meets the needs of the present without compromising the ability of future generations to meet their own needs" (1987). This definition has, in retrospect, become almost iconic for both what it says and, perhaps even more so, for what it doesn't say, a fact that, as Redclift has pointed out, makes the very concept of sustainable development highly polyvocal, bordering on the oxymoronic (2002, 2005).

We will return to the many contradictions, tensions, and problematic invocations of sustainable development later on in this chapter; however, we want to trace the genealogy of the term even further back in time to more clearly align it with sexual health, that is, sex and reproduction, as impacting societal and ecological sustainability.

Sustainable development and its rise to prominence were heralded by its impact within the Earth Summit and the Brundtland Commission, and thus the stage was set for it to become incorporated within public policies across the globe (Grober, 2007; Grober & Cunningham, 2012; Redclift, 1992, 1993, 2002, 2005). However, the genealogy of sustainable development points us even further back in time. In 1980, for instance, the International Union for the Conservation of Nature (IUCN), an association of nation-states, environmental agencies, NGOs, the United Nations Environmental Program (UNEP), and the World Wide Fund for Nature (WWF), published a document titled "World Conservation Strategy: Living Resource Conservation for Sustainable Development"[1] (Grober, 2007, p. 5). In it, the IUCN laid the foundation of a discourse that focused on the *sustainable cultivation* and usage of natural resources to ensure sustainable development. A few years earlier, in 1974, another version of sustainable development was framed by the ecumenical World Council of Churches (WCC) at their world conference in Bucharest titled "Science and Technology for Human Development."[2] Here the WCC used a vocabulary built on a biblical "swords-to-plowshares" rhetoric which was in contrast, perhaps, to the IUCN and Brundtland Commission's rhetoric. At their world conference, the WCC wanted to formulate not only a rhetorical shift in policy and politics, but their aim was also one wherein the ultimate goal might be the formulation of a new socioethical guideline from where nations and individuals could thereafter navigate (Grober, 2007, p. 6). The WCC had for some time before this followed the socioethical line of a "responsible society"; however, in the wake of the 1974 conference, the WCC adopted the notion of working towards a "just and sustainable society" which would be achieved by utilizing the highly biblical term "husbanding" (Grober, 2007, p. 6). A sustainable society could only be achieved, the WCC stated, if the global society acknowledged that "the future will require a husbanding of resources and a reduction of the expectations of global economic growth" (WCC cited in Grober, 2007, p. 6). This line was followed up in the WCC's engagements with the concept of sustainability and sustainable development when

> the WCC decided in 1976 that the "Search for a Just, Participatory and Sustainable Society" would be a major emphasis for the future work of the Council. This in turn led to a 1979 conference on "Faith, Science and the Future" at the Massachusetts Institute of Technology, near Boston in the United States.[3]

It is interesting to note the early involvement of the ecumenical community on the question of sustainable development.

Recent calls have been made to involve and partner with interfaith groups and religious groupings on the road to achieving the SDGs, in particular in the case of HIV/AIDS (Narayanan, 2013; Sidibé, 2016). This has also been the case in relation to, for instance, climate change in the case of the Catholic Church and other institutional forms of religion (Agliardo, 2013; Ashley et al., 2013). From a theoretical point of view, the invocation of a "husbanding" of resources in a sustainable fashion, as witnessed in the rhetoric of the WCC, points us also in the direction of a certain sense of being led, by someone taking charge and sustainably cultivating the land. As is well known by now, the very term "husbandry" is derived from a root form which can be taken to mean either "the care, cultivation, and breeding of crops and animals" or "management and conservation of resources."[4] The etymology of "husbanding" is derived from Middle English and its connection to "husband" in the obsolete sense, "farmer."[5] The usage of husbanding in the rhetoric of the WCC can be connected to a long line of Christian conceptualization of mankind being given custodianship of the planet by God; thus, the extension of this kind of rhetoric into the idea of sustainable development is not only an extension of Christian ethics of care but also a Christian idea of custodianship of the planet and its resources (Kearns, 1996). The link between Christian ethics of ecology and stewardship can perhaps best be discerned in the Earth Bible Project launched in Australia by a group of theologists "located at the Centre for Theology, Science and Culture associated with the Adelaide College of Divinity and Flinders University of South Australia" (Conradie, 2004, p. 123). In the Earth Bible Project, the

> team employs an ideology-critical hermeneutic articulated in six "ecojustice principles" in reading the Bible. These principles seek to come to terms with the pervasive anthropocentrism that has been present in the production of the biblical texts, which is evident in the surface structure of the text and that has distorted the history of interpretation and contemporary reinterpretations of the Bible.
>
> (Conradie, 2004, p. 125)

While we cannot dedicate a full review or background to the Earth Bible Project, suffice it to say that the connection between sustainable development and Christianity within the framework of the Global North has been an important factor in shaping some of the discourses around stewardship and ecology.

While this short passage of the impact and genesis of the concept of sustainable development was filtered through the WCC, the usage of the term "sustainable development" within the WCC was in turn already influenced by how sustainable development had been defined by the now-iconic formulations done by the so-called Club of Rome in 1972 and its publication of the report "Limits to Growth" (Meadows et al., 1972). "Limits to Growth" was a report compiled by a group of scientists led by Dennis and Donella Meadows from MIT. In "Limits to Growth," the Club of Rome called for a "state of global equilibrium" wherein it was searching for a "model output that represents a world system that is: 1. *Sustainable* without sudden and uncontrolled collapse; and 2. capable of satisfying the basic material requirements of all of its people" (Grober, 2007, p. 6).

In invoking the notion of a "sustainable world" which would "satisfy the basic material" needs of all its people, the Club of Rome, in "Limits to Growth," pointed out that the Earth and its resources were finite and that development and growth needed to be framed within a notion of finite resources rather than a framework of ever-increasing growth (Grober & Cunningham, 2012, p. 158). The Club of Rome stated that while the upper limits of the growth potential of the Earth were rather uncertain, one clear fact remained: there was a limit, and to go beyond that limit would have catastrophic consequences (Grober & Cunningham, 2012, p. 158). In arguing for this kind of view, the Club of Rome saw two possible ways of relating to the fact that the earth's resources were finite; the first was to live within the confines of these limits, to accommodate ourselves within what the Club of Rome called the Earth's "ultimate carrying capacity" (Grober & Cunningham, 2012, p. 158). The other way forward was to ignore the limits of the Earth's resources and its carrying capacity and rather bet on humankind's ability to extend them through technology in the future or just "overshoot" the limits, in which case the Club of Rome predicted a catastrophic collapse (Grober & Cunningham, 2012, p. 159). This potential collapse is envisioned as coming about through the depletion of the Earth's non-renewable resources, a leap in population, a subsequent food shortage, and, finally, the Earth's inability to absorb all the pollution put out by increased industrialization. The Club of Rome stated that to avoid this collapse, what was in order was more than just the invention of technological solutions to the issue of creating a world which was sustainable; what was indeed needed was a combination of technical solutions as well as a fundamental change in the global human value system (Grober & Cunningham, 2012, p. 159). This change would, in the future, lead to a conceptualization of growth as something immaterial (Grober & Cunningham, 2012, p. 159), the report argued, for, if not, an ecological and civil collapse would ensue when the ultimate carrying capacity of the Earth was breached.

Roots in forestry

If the Club of Rome hinted at the extension of the concept of sustainable development into the sphere of the immaterial, then the historical genesis of the term was anything but immaterial.

Grober has convincingly argued for the link between the modern concept of sustainable development and the work done on forestry in Germany by Hans Carl von Carlowitz in the 17th century (Grober, 2007; Grober & Cunningham, 2012; von Carlowitz & von Rohr, 1732). The same has been argued by Keith Tribe (Tribe, 1984) and Henry E. Lowood (Lowood, 1990). As Grober states, the term "sustainable development" derives much of its semiotic extensions from the term "sustainable yield," which was, as Grober says, "the Holy Grail" of forestry across Europe and the world for more or less two centuries (Grober, 2007, p. 7; Grober & Cunningham, 2012). When the Club of Rome projected that sustainable development of the future hinged on the extension of growth into the realm of the immaterial and value-based, then the start of the idea of sustainable yield lay in the very practical and material realm of forestry, as envisioned by Carlowitz some 250 years before both the Brundtland Commission and the Club of Rome. The German term that was used by Carlowitz was *nachhaltig*, which in English would be translated fairly literally to "sustainable yield." Carlowitz, in publishing his *Sylvicultura Oeconomica* (von Carlowitz & von Rohr, 1732), had, in turn, two main sources of inspiration for his take on how forestry could be made to be in line with a paradigm of sustainable yielding; one was the work of the Englishman John Evelyn and his *Sylva*, published in 1664 (Evelyn, 2013), and the other the Frenchman Jean Baptiste Colbert's work *Ordonnace* of 1669 (Colbert, 1868; Joubleau & Colbert, 1856). Now what spurred this concern for securing sustainable yields in terms of timber and forestry was a concern in both Germany, France, and England that the increase in mining and the construction of ships were depleting the forests of timber faster than it grew on its own. The essence of this concern about sustained yield forestry can be discerned in the words of the American William A. Duerr, who stated that sustained yield forestry was

> our obligation to our decedents and to stabilize our communities, each generation should sustain its resources at a high level and hand them along undiminished. The sustained yield of timber is an aspect of man's most fundamental need: to sustain life itself.
>
> (Duerr cited in Grober, 2007, p. 7)

Duerr's formulation seems almost uncannily a precursor to the essence of the Brundtland Commission's formulations, as well as the UN SDGs. However, sustainable yield, as it was framed by Carlowitz, Evelyn, and Colbert, was perhaps less metaphysically grounded in an imperative to protect future generations from the consumption of the present generation; rather, they were more practical and even political in nature.

The sudden realization that timber was being consumed at a pace that would prevent it from regrowing fast enough was seen as both a practical issue of resources but also an economical and a political one. In England, the concern that woodlands were vanishing became a matter of national security as the fleet admirals brought the concern to the attention of the Royal Society, as they were highly concerned that they would not have enough timber to continue to produce naval flagships (Grober, 2007, p. 8). Evelyn, for instance, in his *Sylva*, stated that "the late increase of shipping . . . multiplication of glass-works, iron furnaces and the like . . . destructive razing and converting of woods to pasture" (2013, pp. 1, 262) had caused the devastation of the "greatest magazines of wealth and glory of this nation," which had become "epidemical" (2013, p. 270). Evelyn proposed that through his analysis of the destruction of the English woodlands, what was called for was a combination of preservation and restoration of the woodlands: "may such Woods as do remain intire be carefully Preserved, and such as are destroy'd, sedulously Repair'd" (Evelyn cited in Grober, 2007, p. 10). Evelyn fills his book with many practical solutions to the problem of achieving a sustainable yield, one of which was to move the ironworks from Old England to New England, that is, the English colonies in America (Evelyn, 2013, p. 11). Other suggestions that are mentioned would be to divide the land plots used for timber into partitions and only fell trees in one partition each year so as to ensure the trees grow back in time for a new cycle (Evelyn, 2013, p. 11). However, while being very practical and a call to "arise then and plan!" (Evelyn, 2013, p. 279), Evelyn also has a call for sustainable yield to include a concern for subsequent generations.

As Grober states, Evelyn's concern for future generations can be discerned when Evelyn claims that each generation was not born for itself but for posterity (Grober, 2007, p. 11). Evelyn goes on to state that

> men should perpetually be planting, that so posterity might have Trees fit for their service . . . which it is impossible they should have if we thus continue to destroy our Woods, without this providential planting in their stead, and felling what we do cut down with great discretion and regard to the future.
>
> (2013, p. 11)

By citing future generations to come and their need for timber, Evelyn also inserts an ethical paradigm in terms of forestry and sustainable yield. Not only was forestry to be a matter of the present and its industries and politics; rather, the cultivation of the forests became for Evelyn an issue of the future, an issue that needed to be dealt with in such a manner that the needs and ambitions of the present generation did not compromise the needs of future generations. Once again, it is uncannily similar to the wording of the Brundtland Commission in saying that sustainable development should be defined as "development that meets the needs of the present without compromising the ability of the future generations to meet their own needs" (1987).

Across the English Channel, the French also dealt with very similar issues, which were subsequently taken up by King Lois XVI's almighty Intendant des Finances and the secretary of the navy, Jean Baptiste Colbert, in his work on the importance of timber for the French nation. Baptiste argued that timber was a resource that needed to be given a special priority, as it was important for the generation of income tax to the crown, as well as being used in mining and, even more specifically, shipbuilding and naval trade (Grober, 2007, p. 13). Seeing as France was a nation built upon mercantilism (Foucault, 2003, 2007, 2008), ships were crucial in extending trade relations, as well as being key in establishing a navy. To secure a stable, reliable, and long-term supply of timber for this project, Colbert wrote of the need to reverse the current trend of deforestation and called upon France to follow his new forest reforms. What was needed was: to restore income to the treasury from the royal forests, to dispel the fears about a timber shortage, and, finally, to secure enough timber for the shipyards (Grober & Cunningham, 2012, p. 72). The king himself had handwritten a note stating that this could only be achieved by "un bon menage des bois" or good management of the woods (Grober & Cunningham, 2012, p. 72). Colbert designed a set of guiding principles that were meant to both tighten control over the royal forests and reestablish and conserve the forest through measures that were to "reduce the use according to the capacity," or, in French, *la reduction des usasges a leur possibil-lite* (Grober, 2007, p. 14). Practically speaking, Colbert suggested implementing laws and regulations that prohibited vagabonding and starting forest fires as well as reducing grazing areas, reorganizing the timber industry, and tightening control over usage rights to the forests (Sand, 2007). While Colbert's ordnances were highly successful the first ten years after they were set into motion, they were not durable, and by the eve of the French Revolution, France had, as Grober states, fewer woodlands than it had had in 1669 (Grober, 2007, p. 15). However, the lack of a durable and sustained effort to protect the French woodlands should perhaps not be seen as an utter failure. A case in point would be Rousseau, who, inspired by Colbert and traditional forestry methods in his native Swiss mountain home, suggested that there should be a balance between consumption and reproduction in his plan for the development of Corse (Grober, 2007; Rousseau & Chesnais, 2000). This would, of course, also become important for Malthus, who, perhaps more than any other, made the connection between populations, consumption, and reproduction (Malthus, 2018), a point we will return to in connection with the genealogy of the concept of sexual health.

So far, we have looked at the work of a Frenchman, Colbert, and an English-man, Evelyn, but the man who perhaps more than anyone has been seen as a key contributor to the development of the semantic root of sustainable develop-ment was the German Hans Carl von Carlowitz (Grober, 2007; Grober & Cun-ningham, 2012; Lowood, 1990). Carlowitz, head of the mining administration in Saxony, published in 1713 his *Sylvicultura oeconomica* (von Carlowitz & von Rohr, 1732). In it, he argued, over 400 pages, against what he saw as the short-term thinking of people in the timber industry, individuals he regarded as being interested only in making money from the industry. He argued that the devastation of the European forests would lead to a timber crisis that would ruin the silver mining industry, as well as the smelting industry, which would be a tremendous financial crisis (Grober, 2007, p. 18). Carlowitz instead argued that one should practically conserve the forests by implementing energy-saving stoves in houses and the metallurgy industry, as well as searching for new substitutes for timber such as fossil fuels like turf (Grober, 2007, p. 18). His more overarching and conceptually addressed ideas built on the concept that there should be a balance between renewal and cutting of trees in such a way that the timber could be used in perpetuity (Grober, 2007, p. 19). His direct, albeit in this context translated, words connected to achieving this goal read: "how to achieve such conservation and growing of timber that there will be a continual and sustained usage" (Grober, 2007, p. 19; von Carlowitz & von Rohr, 1732). In articulating this idea, Carlow-itz points to an idea that is still with us today in dealing with the UN SDGs: that consumption of resources must balance between meeting the needs of the current world while, on the other hand, also being directed towards a future generation in such a way that the current generation's consumption patterns do not compromise future generations' needs.

Carlowitz thus also combines notions of eco-conservation with those of devel-opment and growth, yet the growth he describes is one that is within the limits of what Evelyn called "ultimate carrying capacity," as we recall from earlier. Carlowitz does not seek to go beyond nature's limits, and, indeed, his inspiration for this is taken both from Evelyn and Colbert but also, as Grober states, from the Lutheran theology of not "acting against nature" (Grober, 2007, p. 20). For Carlowitz, Lutheran theology intersects with a political economy of balancing consumption and conservation; on the one hand, one must cultivate the land in such a way that timber can be used to produce materials for both houses and everyday items and also for the mining and metallurgy industries. On the other hand, one must balance this usage with the conservation of timber so that it can "carry" on in perpetuity. Yet the theological aspect is also key here: recognizing that there is a limit to nature, one must not act against nature, and any lavish, wasteful, and harmful use of nature, a direct over-use, is a ruinous sin which must be avoided (Grober, 2007, p. 20). Once again, we see that conservationism has a long history of intersecting with theology and, in particular here, with Lutheran Christianity. We saw this in the modern example of the WCC and its conservation theology which, as we noted earlier, has also become key in various partnerships in trying to implement the SDGs through local NGOs which are rooted in Christian doctrine. This has been the case in many of the sub-Saharan African initiatives of preventing HIV, for instance, wherein various actors such as President's Emergency Plan for AIDS Relief (PEPFAR) have actively allied themselves with "faith-based NGOs" to deliver faith-based prevention initiatives (Cooper, 2015; Levin, 2014).

Pivoting back to Carlowitz, the influence of Lutheran theology on him also had implications for a more socioethical paradigm in terms of the idea of "sustainable yield." For Carlowitz, a fundamental idea was that sustainable yields were also grounded in the right that everyone had to nourishment and subsistence, even the poor, and the dear *posterity* (Grober, 2007, p. 20). Hence Carlowitz's ideological underpinnings read very much like the Brundtland Commission, as well as the UN SDGs, with their focus on "leaving no one behind" and on future generations. As such, Carlowitz combines what Keith Tribe and Henry Lowood describe as "cameral sciences," that is, practical forestry and mathematics (Lowood, 1990; Tribe, 1984), with what Grober describes as "the contours of a new cultural concept made visible" (2007, p. 20).

After the work of Evelyn, Colbert, and finally Carlowitz, the notion of sustainable yield becomes both part of the cameral sciences and of the Physiocrats and their focus on "a science of governing" or government (Lowood, 1990; Tribe, 1984). It became part and parcel of the increased emphasis on the merger of mathematics and statistics, facts, and figures, with that of the management of the State (Lowood, 1990, p. 317). This can be connected with the rise of what Foucault termed "the rise of biopolitics" (Foucault, 2008), wherein statistics, figures, numbers, and a host of other regimes of gaining a panoptic view of the state were becoming increasingly important for the European states in the 18th century onwards.

Forestry and sustainable yield were part of this new focus, and much of what has been described in the previous in terms of the consumption of timber and the conservation of forests was becoming more and more the problem of reproduction and people. The cameral science of forest management become increasingly dominated by formal regulations, procedures, and the combination between the abstract discipline of mathematics and the practical endeavor of forestry, which in turn gave rise to practical usage and implementation of mathematics in the service of securing sustainable yields of timber (Lowood, 1990, pp. 338–340). This science sought to establish an "equilibrium" between not only consumption and conservation of timber but also, on a more abstract level, between the freedom of the current generation to heed its own needs and the projected needs and growth of future generations to come (Tribe, 1984, p. 276). However, if this short genealogy of the conceptual framework of sustainable development is to be of further use to us in the setting of our focus on the current iteration of sustainability and sexual health, we cannot avoid the connection that this story of sustainable yield has to the problem of the figure of the "population" as it emerged in the late 18th and early 19th centuries.

If Evelyn, Colbert, and Carlowitz highlighted the need for and focus on the potential implications of deforestation and the overconsumption of timber within the political milieu of European states in the 18th century, then the grim report that followed somewhat similar lines of argument concerning the issue of population growth must also be told, if only in brief. Of course, this story starts with none other than Thomas Robert Malthus and his *An Essay on the Principle of Population* (Malthus, 2018). It is by connecting the genealogy of the term "sustainable development" to the work of Malthus that we can draw lines directly to the Club of Rome, then to the Brundtland Commission, and finally to the SDGs' focus on sexual and reproductive health. Ultimately, this focus links a certain notion of sustainable yield with ecology, human reproduction, the state, and the individual to one word: sex.

Connecting sex to population control: the historical intersections between sex and sustainable development

The connection between the genealogy of sustainable development and sex is, of course, deeply connected to the influence of the work of Thomas Robert Malthus and his *An Essay on the Principle of Population*, which was published in 1798 (Malthus, 1888) but went through no less than six revisions and editions. In his work, Malthus responded to what he saw as the naïve and utopic perspectives of his contemporaries William Godwin (Godwin, 2015) and Marquis de Condorcet (Condorcet, 2009) on population growth and its relationship to food production, that is, sustaining the population as it grew. Instead of Godwin's and Condorcet's optimism about the "perfectibility" of the human mind to ever develop and grow, Malthus painted a grim picture of an innate fault within humanity's relationship to nature and the relationship between population growth and sustainment. In response to what Malthus saw as the utopian visions of Godwin and Condorcet, he wrote that

> This natural inequality of the two powers, of population, and production of
> the earth, and that great law of our nature which must constantly keep their

effects equal, form the great difficulty that appears to me insurmountable in the way to the perfectibility of society.

(1999)

For Malthus, there is, as Dean states, an ontological given disequilibrium in the laws of life, that is, between the rate of growth of the population and the rate of growth of its means of subsistence (2015, p. 20). In rather technocratic terms, Malthus postulated that populations grow at a "geometrical" level, while food production grows or rises in an arithmetic ratio (Burgett, 2002, p. 125). This meant that Malthus saw populations growing at an exponential rate, while food and sustenance for said populations grew at a linear rate; thus, built into the onto-logical relationship that any given population had with its natural surroundings was what has been called a "Malthusian trap" (Macfarlane, 2002, 2003) – that is, that population growth will eventually outgrow its sources of food, leading to disastrous outcomes in terms of hunger, civil unrest, and potential collapse of the society in question. Malthus went on to describe this in the following way:

> If the subsistence for man that the earth affords was to be increased every twenty-five years by a quantity equal to what the whole world at present pro-duces, this would allow the power of production in the earth to be unlimited, and its ratio of increase much greater than we can conceive that any possible exertions of mankind could make it. . . . yet still the power of population being a power of a superior order, the increase of the human species can only be kept commensurate to the increase of the means of subsistence by the constant operation of the strong law of necessity acting as a check upon the greater power.
>
> (1999, p. 8)

Already at this juncture, is it possible to see the parallels to the concerns that had plagued Carlowitz, Evelyn, and Colbert; humankind for all of these thinkers balanced on a potential knife's edge, and only through vigilance and continual checks and balances between mankind and nature could mankind thrive both in relationship to natural resources such as timber and coal but also concerning food resources.

Malthus saw, however, potential solutions to this ontological disequilibrium; humans needed to enforce checks and balances upon themselves were they to avoid the tragic outcomes of the trap that lay on the horizon. Some of these checks were almost ontologically hardwired into mankind's relationship to nature; they could be seen as so-called "positive checks," that is, checks that increased death/ mortality rates. Here we can count malnutrition, disease, famine, and war amongst the "positive checks" on a population (Bergthaller, 2018, p. 42). On the other side of the spectrum, we have so-called "preventive checks," that is, checks that were meant to lessen the birth rate within a population. Here we can note celibacy before marriage as one such check, as well as delaying marriage until such a time wherein one could *sustain* a family (Bergthaller, 2018, p. 42). This is where

Malthus becomes not just a theorist of demographics or of reproduction and a certain strain of "sustainable yield" – no, it is here that Malthus also becomes a man who concerns himself with sex and thus theories of sex and sexuality. It is here that reproduction meets sex, it is here that the intimacies and desires of the individual become a matter of the state, and it is here that the sexual lives of the citizens of the state become relevant to the life and health of the state and not just the individual. It should be noted that these kinds of "preventive checks" are still very much part of modern reproductive health discourses: the UN's notion of "too soon, too close and too late" strategy focuses squarely on birth timing, that is, that one should not have children too soon, nor should the spacing be too close, and, finally, one should avoid waiting too long. This is part of the modern and logical extension of what Malthus was focusing on in terms of the preventive checks.

Observe Malthus' statement in the following: "I think I may fairly make two postulata: First, That food is necessary to the existence of man. Secondly, That the passion between the sexes is necessary and will remain in nearly its present state" (cited in McLane, 2013, p. 343). If Deleuze and Guattari wrote in their seminal work *Anti-Oedipus* that there are only desire and the social (Deleuze et al., 2014), then Malthus might be read as stating that there is only desire and food (McLane, 2013, p. 343). Food and desire are part and parcel of the very ontological problem of humanity; the supply of food will, according to Malthus, always be in direct opposition to the driving (sexual) desires of humans. And while reproduction has been the focal term used in describing the Malthusian trap, that is, the relationship between human reproduction and human food production, it is indeed carnal desires which are at stake in Malthus' treatise on the human population. Much ink has been spilled on Malthus' radical formulation of a science of demography and its radical implication for the political economy (Dean, 2015); however, several scholars have also noted Malthus' importance as a scholar of sex and desire, which is intimately if implicitly stated in his work (Bederman, 2008; Burgett, 2002; Folbre, 1992; McLane, 2013; Nicholson, 1990).

It is here, we argue, that the genealogy between a theory of sustainable yield and Malthusian population concerns intersects, or starts to intersect, with the modern history of sustainable development. Going back to Malthus' focus on the "preventive checks," these checks are founded on moral and normative grounds to limit the "great power" asymmetry between the geometric growth of populations and the linear growth of production.

As stated, these checks include celibacy and delaying marriage. What both of these checks have in common is a certain sense of foresight and a directionality towards the future. Much like in the works of Carlowitz, Colbert, and Evelyn, there is a sense of the future, of planning, and of wit that is in play. As McLane states, Malthus' theory is a theory of reproducing bodies, a theory that plays in the subject's ability to envision and plan according to his or her imagination of a future to come wherein it is the subject through these preventive checks that continually battle between his/her desires and the carrying capacity of sustenance around the community of the subject (McLane, 2013, p. 344). Malthus defined these preventive checks as a way of lessening birth rates to lessen the impact of the alleged geometric growth rate upon the linear growth rate of food supplies. Abstinence from sexual intercourse was the only acceptable preventive check upon the desire of the bodies of the people. The sensual passions, as he termed them, needed to be kept in check not just on moral grounds; rather, they threatened what we would have called "the sustainability of the community" and even the nation. For

> the cravings of hunger, the love of liquor, the desire of possessing a beautiful woman, will urge men to actions, of the fatal consequences of which, to the general interest of society, they are perfectly well convinced, even as the very time they commit them. Remove their bodily cravings, and they would not hesitate a moment in determining against such actions.
>
> (Malthus cited in Folbre, 1992, p. 113)

Malthus sees these bodily cravings as being subversive of rational actions, actions that would keep the balance between the growth of human populations, on the one hand, and the growth of food, on the other, in check. Mankind (often here, of course, mediated in the male form), knows better only if there are checks in place to hinder men in accessing or satisfying their carnal desires. If we could remove these desires, then men would "know" that these carnal desires were wrong on moral grounds but also within the setting of a Malthusian economy of sustainability.

Malthus' focus on sex warrants more elaboration, as it is important to follow this lead in our genealogy of the connection between sustainability and sexual health. Given that Malthus saw food and "the passion between the sexes" as key in his political economy, this also meant coming to terms with how to check these passions. As stated, celibacy was one such preventive check, as was delaying one's time of marriage. However, these checks were not only practically based, but they also came as responses to the work of the aforementioned Godwin and Condorcet, as well as to the work of David Hume. In Hume's 1752 *Of the Populousness of Ancient Nations* (1977), Hume had argued for the lifting of all constraints on the "desire and power of generation," and this recommendation followed from the premise that it seemed "natural" to Hume that "wherever there are the most happiness and virtue and the wisest institutions, there will also be the most people" (Burgett, 2002, p. 126). Following this, both Godwin and Condorcet had argued that while it was true that periodical diseases and wars will ensue when the number of people exceeds the means of subsistence, they both nevertheless also argued that the future of mankind was bright, due in large part to the "perfectibility" of humanity's rational thinking and the advancement of knowledge (Burgett, 2002, p. 126). Godwin connected this problematic to the issue of sex and desire when he stated that man's desire would atrophy as he marched into his perfectible future; indeed, as Godwin says, this future is a future wherein "men will probably cease to propagate. The whole will be a people of men, not of children. Generation will not succeed generation, nor truth have, to a certain degree, to recommend her career every thirty years" (1820, p. 776).

In contrast to this, Malthus responded to Godwin's speculation of the atrophy of the "passion between the sexes" in the following manner: "towards the extension of the passion between the sexes, no progress whatsoever has hitherto been made. It appears to exist in as much force at present as it did two thousand or four thousand years ago" (cited in McLane, 2013, p. 349). Malthus' focus, on the surface of it, seems to be that of solving the ontological trap that belies mankind's relationship to its surrounding natural environment in such a way as to make this embedded disequilibrium into a sustainable equilibrium. However, this is as much about sex as it is about food. In an interesting juxtaposition, Maureen McLane states that Aristotle defined man as the political animal, Marx analyzed man as the laboring animal, Raymond Williams constructed man as the communicating animal, and Malthus can be seen to propose man as a desiring being (McLane, 2013, p. 349). Mankind desires, in Malthus, food and sex, yet the availability of each of the two is contingent upon one another. Food and sex, that is, reproductive sex, are entangled in such a fashion that the two desires are never fully separated from each other. Reproductive sex must heed the ecological frame in which it is located, and, in turn, food, or sustenance, is contingent upon the number of people within the ecological network. The danger of the "Malthusian trap" lies within every individual body and its desires; it is in a sense the "uncontrollability of its reproductive capacities as the inescapable premise and central problem of his social and political theory" (Burgett, 2002, p. 126). As Thomas Laqueur chimes in: "Malthus insists on the absolute primacy of the sexual body in the political economy" (cited in Stanton, 1992, p. 202).

A quick summary here would lead us to state that while the work of Carlowitz, Colbert, and Evelyn was fundamental for the epistemological possibility of the very concept of "sustainable development" and thus the SDGs, the work of Malthus and in turn his contemporaries became intimately connected to a sort of parallel discourse of "sustained yield" and ultimate carrying capacity. However, for Malthus, Godwin, Condorcet, and even Jeremy Bentham, it was, implicitly or explicitly, sex that was the great problematic. Reproductive sex needed to be controlled and not just based on religious and moral grounds; rather, it needed to be checked by preventive measures so that society at large could sustain itself. This would be taken up with full effect in the 1960s and 1970s, as we will shortly show; however, it is worth noting how sex becomes problematic for the state, and indeed the state's very survival hinges upon solving the "Malthusian trap," which turns out to be, in the final analysis, a problem of desire.

While for Malthus, the issues of population control and sex were key, this would also become important within a framework for the development of a moral economy of disease, infirmary, and sexuality when it was coupled with not only reproductive sex but indeed sex as a vector for diseases. The link between Malthusian concerns about population control and sustainability and sex can be seen in the preoccupation with certain diseases and, of course, sex and sexuality. Reproductive health and sex were the objects of Malthus, yet the concept of sexual health would not emerge until the 1970s. It is to the concept of sexual health that the next chapter will be dedicated.

Notes

1 See the full document online here. https://portals.iucn.org/library/sites/library/files/ documents/WCS-004.pdf
2 See the WCC's press center online and its statements on sustainable development. www.oik- oumene.org/en/press-centre/news/sustainability-and-environment-how-the-ecumenical- movement-helped-mobilize-ecology-protest-in-east-germany
3 Ibid.
4 See the Oxford English Dictionary for its meaning as well as its etymology. https:// en.oxforddictionaries.com/definition/husbandry
5 Ibid.

References

Agliardo, M. (2013). The US Catholic response to climate change. *How the World's Reli- gions Are Responding to Climate Change: Social Scientific Investigations, 12*, 174.
Ashley, M., Baur, M., Brinkman, J. T., Cloutier, D., Dolcich-Ashley, A., Groppe, E., Hefel- finger, S. G., Irwin, K. W., Kettler, D., Peppard, C. Z., Unabali, B., Vallery, J., Warner, K. D., & Peppard, C. Z. (2013). *Environmental justice and climate change: Assessing Pope Benedict XVI's ecological vision for the Catholic Church in the United States.* Lexington Books.
Bederman, G. (2008). Sex, scandal, satire, and population in 1798: Revisiting Malthus's first essay. *Journal of British Studies, 47*(4), 768–795.
Bergthaller, H. (2018). *Malthusian biopolitics, ecological immunity, and the anthropocene.* National Chung-Hsing University.
Brundtland Commission. (1987). *World Commission on Environment and Development: Our common future.* Oxford University Press.
Burgett, B. (2002). Between speculation and population: The problem of "sex" in our long eighteenth century. *Early American Literature, 37*(1), 119–153.
Colbert, J. B. (1868). *Lettres, instructions et mémoires* (vol. 5). Imprimerie Impériale.
Condorcet, A. N. (2009). *Outlines of a historical view of the progress of the human mind.* G. Langer, Lulu. com.
Conradie, E. M. (2004). Towards an ecological biblical hermeneutics: A review essay on the earth Bible project. *Scriptura: Journal for Contextual Hermeneutics in Southern Africa, 85*(1), 123–135.
Cooper, M. (2015). The theology of emergency: Welfare reform, US foreign aid, and the faith-based initiative. *Theory, Culture & Society, 32*(2), 53–77.
Dean, M. (2015). The Malthus effect: Population and the liberal government of life. *Econ- omy and Society, 44*(1), 18–39.
Deleuze, G., Guattari, F., & Massumi, B. (2014). *A thousand plateaus: Capitalism and schizophrenia.* University of Minnesota Press.
Earth Summit. (1992). *The United Nations program for action from Rio.* Agenda 21. https://sustainabledevelopment.un.org/outcomedocuments/agenda21
Evelyn, J. (2013). *Sylva, or, a discourse of forest trees: With an essay on the life and works of the author* (vol. 1). Cambridge University Press.
Folbre, N. (1992). "The improper arts": Sex in classical political economy. *Population and Development Review*, 105–121.
Foucault, M. (2003). *"Society Must Be Defended": Lectures at the Collège de France, 1975–1976* (vol. 1). Macmillan.

Foucault, M. (2007). *Security, territory, population: Lectures at the Collège de France, 1977–78.* Springer.

Foucault, M. (2008). *The birth of biopolitics: Lectures at the Collège de France, 1978–1979.* Springer.

Godwin, W. (1820). *Of population: An enquiry concerning the power of increase in the numbers of mankind, being an answer to Mr. Malthus's essay on that subject.* Printed for Longman, Hurst, Rees, Orme, and Brown.

Godwin, W. (2015). *Inquiry concerning political justice: And its influence on morals and happiness.* Penguin Books.

Grober, U. (2007). *Deep roots – A conceptual history of sustainable development (Nachhaltigkeit).* Discussion Papers, Presidential Department P 2007-002. Social Science Center.

Grober, U., & Cunningham, R. (2012). *Sustainability: A cultural history.* Green Books.

Hume, D. (1977). On the populousness of ancient nations. *Population and Development Review, 3*(3), 323–329.

Joubleau, F., & Colbert, J. B. (1856). *Etudes sur Colbert ou exposition du système d'économie politique suivi en France de 1661 à 1683.* Guillaumin.

Kearns, L. (1996). Saving the creation: Christian environmentalism in the United States. *Sociology of Religion, 57*(1), 55–70.

Levin, J. (2014). Faith-based initiatives in health promotion: History, challenges, and current partnerships. *American Journal of Health Promotion, 28*(3), 139–141.

Lowood, H. E. (1990). The calculating forester: Quantification, cameral science, and the emergence of scientific forestry management in Germany. *The Quantifying Spirit in the 18th Century, 11,* 315–342.

Macfarlane, A. (2002). *The savage wars of peace: England, Japan, and the Malthusian trap.* Springer.

Macfarlane, A. (2003). The Malthusian trap. In *The savage wars of peace* (pp. 11–24). Springer.

Malthus, T. R. (1888). *An essay on the principle of population: Or, a view of its past and present effects on human happiness.* Reeves & Turner.

Malthus, T. R. (1999). *Oxford world's classics.* Oxford University Press.

Malthus, T. R. (2018). An essay on the principle of population as it affects the future improvement of society. In *The economics of population* (pp. 41–50). Routledge.

McLane, M. N. (2013). Malthus our contemporary?: Toward a political economy of sex. *Studies in Romanticism, 52*(3), 337–362.

Meadows, D. H., Meadows, D. H., Randers, J., & Behrens III, W. W. (1972). *The limits to growth: A report to the Club of Rome.* Universe Books.

Narayanan, Y. (2013). Religion and sustainable development: Analysing the connections. *Sustainable Development, 21*(2), 131–139.

Nicholson, M. (1990). The eleventh commandment: Sex and spirit in Wollstonecraft and Malthus. *Journal of the History of Ideas,* 401–421.

Redclift, M. (1992). The meaning of sustainable development. *Geoforum, 23*(3), 395–403.

Redclift, M. (1993). Sustainable development: Needs, values, rights. *Environmental Values,* 3–20.

Redclift, M. (2002). *Sustainable development: Exploring the contradictions.* Routledge.

Redclift, M. (2005). Sustainable development (1987–2005): An oxymoron comes of age. *Sustainable Development, 13*(4), 212–227.

Rousseau, J. J., & Chesnais, R. (2000). *Projet de constitution pour la Corse.* Nautilus.

Sand, P. H. (2007). Sustainable development – Of forests, ships, and law. *Environmental Law and Policy Review*, *37*, 202.

Sidibé, M. (2016). Religion and sustainable development. *Review of Faith and International Affairs*, *14*(3). Taylor & Francis.

Stanton, D. C. (1992). *Discourses of sexuality: From Aristotle to AIDS*. University of Michigan Press.

Tribe, K. (1984). Cameralism and the science of government. *The Journal of Modern History*, *56*(2), 263–284.

von Carlowitz, H. C., & von Rohr, J. B. (1732). *Sylvicultura oeconomica*.

3 The genealogy of the concept of sexual health

In this chapter, we will shed light on a few important aspects that impacted the concept of sexual health. We will specifically focus on the launch of the document *Promotion of Sexual Health: Recommendations for Action*, which was produced by the Pan American Health Organization (PAHO) and the WHO (Pan American Health Organization, 2000). Another key document that emerged around the same time and which has heavily influenced the current definition of sexual health was the US surgeon general's *Call to Action to Promote Sexual Health and Responsible Sexual Behavior* (Satcher, 2001). However, we need to go back to the first usage of "sexual health" by the WHO in 1975 to lay out the history of the term and the different meanings the term has had throughout the years. This genealogy has implications for how sexual health is now being refracted through the prism of sustainability. While the previous chapter explored the genealogy of sustainability as a condition of the possibility for sexual health, this chapter has the opposite objective: we will show how the growth of sexual health has implications for the current conception of sexual health. Sustainability, through the lineage of the Malthusian focus on the relationship between the human population on the one hand and natural resources on the other, was always also preoccupied with human reproduction and thus sexuality and sex. As such, sustainability and sexual health are in a way linked. They are linked through a balancing act wherein sexuality and, in extension to this, sexual health exist in a tension-filled space between, on the one hand, vitality and life, and, on the other hand, death and entropy. Sexuality has the power to introduce new vitality into the world through reproduction, but at the same time, it is also the site of potential danger, in terms of illnesses but also overpopulation. It is here that sustainability thinking comes into play, and it is also here that Malthus becomes actualized, as we saw in the prior chapter. In this chapter, we will map how the concept of sexual health has emerged since 1975 and how it has more and more come to take on the colors of explicit sustainability thinking.

More specifically, we will sketch out how the concept of sexual health and, to a certain degree, sexual rights have come to be part and parcel of the SDG goals as well as being epistemologically connected to sustainability and thus also to the Malthusian concern of population and sex.

The WHO included sexual health as an official concept within a statement on the term back in 1975 in its report of *Education and Treatment in Human Sexuality: The Training of Health Professionals* (WHO, 1975). Scholars in the field have loosely agreed that before this statement, sexual health had been researched through a reading that focused mostly on sexual pathology in various forms, be it sexually transmitted infections (STIs), unwanted sexual behavior, sexual identity, or sexualized violence and abuse (Giami, 2002; Sandfort & Ehrhardt, 2004). With the WHO statement on sexual health in 1975, the focus was moved from pathology to an understanding of sexuality and sex more interconnected to the concept of health. The WHO's definition of sexual health has since 1975 gone through some revisions, and the latest definition is to be found in the WHO's report *Defining Sexual Health. Report of a Technical Consultation on Sexual Health* from 2002, which has subsequently been adopted in several other reports from the WHO and other national plans concerning sexual health (Public Health England, 2015; WHO, 2016). The current definition of sexual health reads as follows:

> Sexual health is a state of physical, emotional, mental, and social well-being in relation to sexuality; it is not merely the absence of disease, dysfunction, or infirmity. Sexual health requires a positive and respectful approach to sexuality and sexual relationships, as well as the possibility of having pleasurable and safe sexual experiences, free of coercion, discrimination, and violence. For sexual health to be attained and maintained, the sexual rights of all persons must be respected, protected, and fulfilled.
>
> (WHO, 2002)

What is striking with the WHO's definition is its focus on health and rights and the absence of specific pathological focuses in a holistic definition that even includes pleasure. While the WHO is an important actor when it comes to providing a conceptual definition and framework for the term "sexual health," it is not the only important actor that has been part of the proliferation of conceptual definitions of sexual health. Edwards and Coleman, for instance, point to the Pan American Health Organization's declaration in 2001 as another key text in the proliferation of the concept of sexual health (2004, p. 190). Edwards and Coleman further identify the *US Surgeon General's Report on Sexual Health* from 2001 and the *National Strategy for Sexual Health and HIV*, also from 2001, as key texts that provide both a conceptual grounding for the term and an important bedrock for various organizations, states, and institutions to work with and look at the sexual health of their people (2004, p. 190). Edwards and Coleman's views are shared in part by Epstein and Mamo (2017) and Sandfort and Ehrhardt (2004), and in an earlier, but important, article, Giami also see these texts as foundational for the proliferation of sexual health as a public health issue to be addressed (2002). Since then, several other publications have been published, among them The Lancet series in sexual health, which is in collaboration with the WHO; the European Regional Office of the WHO and its report on sexual health and sustainability (WHO, 2016); and the English report on sexual health and HIV from

2015 (Public Health England, 2015). As such, the very term "sexual health" has had a rapid and prolific spread across a diverse set of discourses and fields, which makes its potential impact both great and probably also unpredictable due to its polyvalence.

Sexual health and the World Health Organization: a beginning

The 1975 definition of sexual health as it emerged in the WHO document *Education and Treatment in Human Sexuality: The Training of Health Professionals* reads as follows:

> Sexual health is the integration of the somatic, emotional, intellectual, and social aspects of sexual being, in ways that are positively enriching and that enhance personality, communication, and love. Thus, the notion of sexual health implies a positive approach to human sexuality, and the purpose of sexual health care should be the enhancement of life and personal relationships and not merely counseling and care related to procreation or sexuality transmitted diseases.
>
> (WHO, 1975, p. 41)

This initial definition, made in 1975, differs in several ways from the 2002 WHO definition, yet it does open up from a more holistic definition of sexual health, in that the 1975 definition moves away from a focus that is only limited to pathologies of STIs or reproduction. The definition, much like that of 2002, is much more positive, and the emphasis is placed on the positive aspects of sexuality through the inclusion of love and personal development. In this way, this 1975 definition also introduces a separation, or at least the possibility of separation, between sexuality and reproduction, a key component of the 1975 definition. As Giami states in his analysis of the 1975 introduction of the term "sexual health":

> The authors of the report defended the general principle of keeping erotic sexual activity autonomous and separate from reproductive sexuality, family planning, and the prevention of sexually transmitted diseases; however, for practical and organizational purposes, they proposed including sexual health intervention in the framework of existing reproductive health interventions.
>
> (2002, p. 11)

Up until the 1975 definition, sexuality and sex within the lexicon of health had mainly been linked to either reproduction or diseases and disease prevention. These, in turn, had a long history of being objects of moral and moralizing discourses on topics such as childbirth outside of wedlock, prostitution and the spread of STIs, and, as seen in the work of Malthus, the moral imperative to have children at a time in one's life when one could afford to feed and take care of the child.

With the 1975 definition, the focus is moved subtly onto the possibility of framing sexual "health" directly within sexuality and not any somatic notion of pathology or reproduction, something which can be discerned when the WHO report states that "Nevertheless, in certain situations, sexuality programs could also be developed outside this context [STI pathology, and reproduction] because of the connotations of birth control" (1975, p. 44). However, as is noted by Giami again, in terms of addressing sexual health, the 1975 definition, for all its holistic focus, nevertheless is firmly embedded within a biomedical and somatic understanding of the many etiologies of different sexual pathologies and disorders; psychological and relational factors, which are now seen as key in developing and fostering sexual health, are omitted in the WHO's rundown of various sexual disorders (2002, p. 11). In this fashion, the 1975 definition still seems to rest on a firm understanding of "healthy sexual health" as being cemented in what is a satisfactory somatic level of health. The 1975 definition also lacked a focus on "sexual rights," an issue that has become key in the newer frameworks of sexual health, as well as being of key importance within the SDG framework, a fact we will come back to later in this book. The 1975 definition, however, was key in opening up a more positive approach to sexuality within public health discourse, though this would be met with some modifications as the HIV/AIDS epidemic emerged in the early 1980s and reached its peak in the Global North in the mid- to late 1990s.

As such, in 1987, the WHO Regional Office released a paper titled "Concepts of Sexual Health: Report of a Working Group" (WHO, 1987). While this report emerged amid the HIV/AIDS epidemic as it was raging, this report, in particular, was not intended to be a public health report; rather, it was seen as a document in which the WHO explored whether there was a "need for a separate sub-category of 'sexual health' and questioned whether a definition of sexual health would be medical, moral, social or psychological" (WHO, 1987, p. 1). As such, the report, as Lottes has remarked, never fully took up the space that the 1975 document did nor any of the subsequent iterations of the term "sexual health" (2000). However, for our purposes here in charting out the history of the term "sexual health," it is worth noting that the document had a rather strong focus on the conceptual *difficulties* of defining what the term "sexual health" could and should come to mean within the WHO lexicon. The difficulty with the term, it was stated, was that "sexual health is not a scientific concept. Concepts of sexual health are related to culture and time and express values and norms of the society of which they come" (WHO, 1987, p. 2). This is in stark contrast to the many sexual health strategies that have been rolled out in the aftermath of the SDGs, wherein, as we shall see later on, there is a strong focus on *evidence-based medical interventions*. For the authors of the 1987 WHO report, sexual health has not only a holistic focus, as in the 1975 definition, it also has a strong *culturalist* and social constructivist veneer. In the 1987 WHO document, the framing of sexual health is less about the holistic and universal attributes that the 1975 definition provided; rather, the authors expressed concerns that there was a danger that the concept of sexual health would end up establishing a norm for sexual health, that a definition of sexual health would become normative and restrictive, and, finally, that there was already an implicit concept of sexual health in all services and education related to sexuality (Giami, 2002, p. 14). This offers an interesting contrast to the 1975 definition and report in that the 1975 report offered a holistic, universal, and research-based call for more research on sexuality and sex, while the 1987 report could be seen as a contrast to this with its hesitant remarks about the "unscientific" nature of sexual health, the many problems it saw in terms of the contextual nature of the term, and the many risks that might be encountered if it were to establish a sexual health framework.

On a more positive note, the 1987 report did note that

the goals of policies, programs, and services relating to sexuality are not that they achieve a measurable level of "sexual health" in the population, but that they enable individuals to meet their needs in the area of sexuality and enable them to have the personal resources to deal with problems and difficulties that arise.

(WHO, 1987, p. 4)

This is also a strong contrast to the many current strategies and services within the field of sexual health services and policies, which are more and more predicated upon "governance through indicators," that is, counting devices which offer surveillance data as well as data which is meant to target areas within sexual health services that are lacking or in need of more resources. A case in point here would be that indicators on HIV/AIDS prevention (UNAIDS, 2019) but also indicators on sexual dysfunction; reproductive data such as abortions, unplanned pregnancies, access to contraception, STI prevalence, and incident rates; and even indicators on sexual rights have come to be included in a great many national and international sexual health strategies and reports, such as in England (Department of Health, England, 2013; Public Health England, 2015), Ireland, Norway (Ministry of Health and Care Services Norway, 2017), France, and Demark. Even the WHO Regional Office Europe's current sexual health plan specifically aimed at achieving the UN's SDGs offers a plethora of indicators that are meant to do exactly what the 1987 report did not want: to achieve measurable levels of "sexual health" (WHO, 2016).

Giami explains the contrasting views between the 1975 report, which was predicated upon a call for more research on sexuality, and, on the other hand, the 1987 report, with its focus and cautious outlook on the normative potentials for sexual health and the current drive towards indicators and metrics under the UN's SDG framework by stating that the 1987 report was "predicated on an individualistic approach to sexual issues, considering that every individual is unique according to his/her needs and expectations" (2002, p. 15). This was in turn framed within a vocabulary that sexuality and sex were seen as being contingent upon the many meanings attributed to sexuality within different cultural and religious contexts around the world. As such, the 1987 report differed sharply from the 1975 report, which strongly opposed religious and cultural issues and saw these as "obstacles" to achieving sexual health. The 1987 report specifically stated that the term "sexual health" should consider the cultural meanings and religious meanings attributed to sexuality; in fact, these issues deserved respect and understanding, according to the 1987 report (WHO, 1987, p. 12). On a more general level, the contrasting views between the 1975 report, the 1987 report, and the current 2016 report offer a tri-part contrast which nevertheless is part of the complex semantic genealogy of the concept of sexual health; the 1987 report states, in contrast to the 1975 report, that sexual health policies should be implemented alongside existing values and beliefs rather than against them, as the 1975 report seemed to state (Giami, 2002, p. 15). The 2016 definition of the WHO's sexual health action plan, on the other hand, offers a third contrast, with its reliance on sexual rights, which is omitted in the 1975 report and the 1987 version, anchored more in line with local cultural values. In the 2016 report, these rights are universal and not linked to local values and beliefs. The 1987 report was unusually concerned that rights and norms connected to the concept of sexual health would end up perpetuating the "values and preferences of middle-class white people" (Giami, 2002, p. 15), a fact that meant that the 1987 report was highly critical of implementing a universal and normative definition of sexual health.

While the 1975 call for a universal, holistic, and science-based concept of sexual health meant that the 1975 WHO document railed against the many misconceptions, taboos, and religious and cultural beliefs surrounding sexuality and sex, the 1987 document went a long way in doing the opposite; instead of highlighting the need for a scientifically accurate, universal definition of sexual health, the 1987 WHO document stated that, "Many health professionals do not know taboos, religious and health beliefs and cultural factors generally. . . . Instead of viewing them as acceptably different, the professional may regard them as ignorant and superstitious. There is a danger of stereotyping" (p. 16). Whereas the 1975 and 2002 WHO definitions of sexual health purported that sexual health should be holistic, based on science and, in the 2002 version, on sexual rights, the 1987 document did two things: first, it focused mostly on the cultural and social issues that affect individual behavior rather than on clinical and pathological aspects of sexual health, as Giami states (2002, p. 16). As such, the 1987 document is an outlier in that the definition provided and the purposes it seeks to establish are not focused on pathology and the biomedical aspects of sexual health; rather, it seeks to establish the complexity of the term "sexual health" in that sexuality itself is seen in the document as relative to the historical and contextual spaces in which it is embedded.

Second, this leads to a form of relativism that seeks to avoid becoming restrictive and normative, which makes the very term "sexual health" polyphonic, which we claim is also part of why the term "sexual health" has come to inhabit a linguistic space where it can be utilized in a vast array of settings, a point we will come back to later in this book. The authors of the 1987 report can be seen as wanting to close the gap between "individual needs and the necessities required for sexual health" (Giami, 2002, p. 16) while at the same time not impeding or restricting local meaning – making sexuality lean heavily on a rights-based framework which also saw evidence-based policies and medical advice as key in establishing what sexual health can and should be, in the manner that the 1975 document sought to do, or as in the 2002 version.

The 1975 definition, as such, with its universal ambitions, holistic take on sexual health, and push for a more scientific approach to sexual health can be seen as part of an effort to not only make sexuality more scientific but also to medicalize it, as many have argued for (Giami & Perrey, 2012). By arguing for a universal and scientific approach to sexual health and subsequently sexuality, the 1975 definition, while being holistic in nature, can also be seen to create a medicalization of sexuality, which relied on a host of disciplinary knowledge-producing groups and institutions. The question that now must be raised is: What kind of knowledge regime are we seeing the contours of in terms of the link between sustainable development, sexual health, and population/state tensions? While we will analyze this in much more detail later on in this book, we cannot skip one of the most important moments in the genealogy of the concept of sexual health which emerged in the early 2000s. As such, we need to shed some light on the important aspects that came into development with the launch of the document *Promotion of Sexual Health: Recommendations for Action* which was produced by the PAHO and the WHO (Pan American Health Organization, 2000). Another key document that emerged around the same time and which would heavily influence the current definition of sexual health was the US surgeon general's *Call to Action to Promote Sexual Health and Responsible Sexual Behavior* (Satcher, 2001). Both of these are important for us in establishing both the genealogy of the term "sexual health" as it has emerged in the public health lexicon but more so because these two action plans also introduced the issue of responsibility and rights, something which the 1975 and 1987 documents did not approach. Risk, responsibility, and rights are key in that these three concepts are also highlighted in the current push for sexual health as it is framed in the SDG framework, and, as such, a short analysis of these two action plans will help to better understand the current definition and framework of sexual health as it is framed within the Agenda 2030 setting.

Buildup to the Sustainable Development Goals: sexual health in the 2000s

We can start with the PAHO Action Plan, which was produced in 2000 in a joint effort between PAHO, WHO, and World Association of Sexologists (WAS). It is interesting to note that the document was produced by this tri-part cooperation between one regional health organization, one global organization, and one organization made up of professionals working in the field of sexology. The document is an example of the increasing professionalization of sexual health and, in turn, the medicalization of sex and sexuality. In the case of the PAHO Action Plan, it is clear that the strong influence that WAS had in the making of the Action Plan can be discerned through the strong focus it had on not only on reproduction but sexuality proper. The reason this is interesting and an indicator of the professionalization and power of sexology lies in the fact that the separation of reproduction and sexuality points to boundary drawing between sexologists and gynecologists/obstetricians, all of them experts within closely related domains. Yet the separation between sexual health and reproductive health as envisioned in the Action

Plan could be taken, as Giami says, a sign of the ongoing professionalization of sexology as a discipline (2002, p. 16), as well as the ongoing disciplinary boundary drawing between the field of sexology and other, more traditional medical fields such as gynecology and even psychiatry. In short, the problematization of sexuality and health when linked into the compound term "sexual health" has led to an immense professionalization around the issue of human sexuality.

Comparing the PAHO 2000 document to the 1975 and 1987 WHO documents, there is a clear change in the language used in terms of how sexual health is framed; there is, for one, a clear usage of science as a frame of reference. Whereas the 1975 and 1987 documents had *no* scientific references, the PAHO Action Plan has 65 references that cite work done in English and Spanish (2000, pp. 49–56). To cite is, as we know, a characteristic of academic writing to ensure transparency, to state where we found our sources, and to show whom we argue against. However, it is also a specific form of *professional writing*, of framing the content of what we write in such a way that the reader of the document understands what genre it is and also of stating a claim to, in this case, scientific authority. The PAHO Action Plan already differs here from the previous two WHO documents in that it firmly leans on the authority of prior research on sexuality and sexual health, and, as Giami notes, this sort of citation practice is a good illustration of the ongoing reinforcement of the scientific basis of sexology (2002, p. 16).

The entire Action Plan starts by laying bare eight "rationales" for its production, and amongst these eight are

> advances in knowledge about different aspects of human sexuality. This has been achieved through theoretical inquiry, biomedical, psychological, sociological and anthropological research, epidemiological surveillance, and clinical work – that have contributed to the development of an extremely complex field, transcending each of the individual disciplines it encompasses.
>
> (Pan American Health Organization, 2000, p. 2)

In this rationale, sexology is implicitly highlighted as representing an area of expertise. However, the Action Plan also highlights that the field of sexology has developed in tandem with twenty-five years of research on sex and developments in evidence-based medicine, as well as developments in the field of pharmacological drugs targeting sexual dysfunction (Pan American Health Organization, 2000). As such, the Action Plan departs from the 1987 documents while perhaps highlighting more so the 1975 vision of an evidence-based sexual health paradigm which also introduces a much stronger focus on responsibility and rights.

Establishing connections between sex, sexuality, health, responsibility, and rights

The PAHO Action Plan is the first of the sexual health documents which firmly establishes a connection between the concepts of sex, sexuality, health, and responsibilities and rights. First of all, the Action Plan establishes a strong focus on the uniqueness of its definition of human sexuality:

> Previous WHO consultations either did not define human sexuality or offered imprecise concepts. As defined here, sexuality refers to the additional components of our sexual nature (the human characteristic of being sexed). The human capacity of understanding and ascribing meanings both symbolic and concrete, to experiences and concepts, are the bonding forces of sexuality. There is general agreement in the literature that sexuality refers to the individual and social meanings of sex, in addition to the biological aspects of sex.
>
> (Pan American Health Organization, 2000, p. 9)

It also goes on to link this definition of sexuality to health through the following definition of sexual health proper:

> Sexual health is the experience of the ongoing process of physical, psychological, and socio-cultural well-being related to sexuality. Sexual health is evidenced in the *free* and *responsible* expressions of sexual capabilities that foster harmonious personal and social wellness, enriching individual and social life. It is not merely the absence of dysfunction, disease, and/or infirmity. For Sexual Health to be attained and maintained the *sexual rights* of all people must be recognized and upheld.
>
> (our italics, Pan American Health Organization, 2000, p. 6)

As we see in the previous, the PAHO declaration introduces the notion that sexual health is something that goes beyond the somatic and biomedical and is rather a holistic entity which is something to be carried out freely yet in a responsible fashion. This tension will come back to haunt the term later on and will become particularly influential within the SDG framework of sexual health and sustainability. Second, the definition provided here also is the first time sexual health is embedded within a rights perspective, a fact that will come to dominate sexual and reproductive health within the SDG framework. The tension between, on the one hand, free sexuality and, on the other hand, an obligation to also act responsibly and follow a rights perspective sets the table for a concept that, as Epstein and Mamo have shown, is highly polyvalent and has come to be used across several sectors of public health but also other state initiatives (2017). This polyvalent nature of sexual health is even picked up by the authors of the PAHO Action Plan, as they state that

> Historically, different groups have used the term "Sexual Health" to mean different things. For some, the term has been used as a euphemism for information on sexually transmitted infections; for others, it has been used to promote a narrow approach to education on reproduction. It should be clear from this definition that in this document, a comprehensive meaning of the concept is proposed.
>
> (Pan American Health Organization, 2000, p. 9)

The authors of the PAHO definition see this polyvalence as something that they need to clarify and thus clearly define; ambiguity and the polyvocal nature of the term are here shunned. The "expert working group agreed that establishing a definition of sexual health is both possible and desirable provided that the definition is derived from, and embodies the concept of sexual rights" (Pan American Health Organization, 2000, p. 10). This last point demonstrates how important a rights-based framework was for the PAHO, the WHO, and WAS; without this framework, the whole concept of sexual health seems to collapse.

Balancing freedom, responsibility, and rights

The definition of such a concept of sexual health seems to be a form of hybrid between the 1975 science and holistic definition of the term and the 1987 version, with its cautious reminders that sexuality is also embedded within sociocultural networks of meaning. However, with the introduction of a rights-based framework, sexual health also becomes something that the subject has a *right* to have, not only something that can be thought of as a part of one's health. This definition also paves the way for a sexual health concept that has to balance freedom, responsibility, and rights. This, in turn, as Giami states, makes the field of sexual health much more clearly defined in terms of mutual responsibility between the individual and the collective (2002, p. 17). While the PAHO definition is tied to the ideals of the 1975 version of the term, the universal tendencies in the 1975 version are set in flux, as we have seen, by the PAHO's reliance on and usage of the term "value(s)" or "systems of values." This phrasing indicates that sexual health is embedded in a plurality of systems that generate value, which could be called "cultures" or systems of beliefs. While the 1975 definition strongly opposed such wording and saw them more as *obstacles* to achieving sexual health, the PAHO's version seems less critical of the notion of a plurality of contexts wherein sexual health emerges. However, the PAHO found a way to circumscribe the troublesome notion of relativism that the 1987 definition found itself in; rather than proposing a universal, and mainly Western, definition of sexual health, the PAHO linked sexual health to a rights perspective, as we have seen.

This rights perspective was not just any framework; the PAHO directly linked these rights to the UN's Universal Human Rights Declaration by highlighting that

> The recognition of sexual rights is evolving. Human rights are those principles that are universally perceived as protecting human dignity while promoting justice, equality, liberty, and life. Since the protection of health is a basic human right, it follows that sexual health involves sexual rights.
>
> (2000, p. 10)

Furthermore, it stated that "Human rights are above cultural values. If a particular culture has a practice that contravenes a human right, the cultural value should be changed, as in the case of the cultural practice of female genital mutilation" (Pan American Health Organization, 2000, p. 10).

By linking sexual health to the WHO's definition of health as a human right and then framing sexual health as being intrinsically linked to sexual rights, this, as we see, shapes an entire rhetorical movement which proposes that sexual health as such is indeed a human right and that while they do acknowledge the many localized variations of sexual health, the values that inform them, and the cultures that produce variations on sexual health and sexuality, the PAHO definition firmly establishes a clear overarching and normative level, which is the UN's human rights framework.

If health is viewed through the "rights to health," as seen in the work of the influential figure of Jonathan Mann (Mann et al., 1994), who firmly set the agenda that health was to become one of the fundamental values of "social life and one of the main criteria for evaluating institutions and political and ideological systems," as Giami notes (2002, p. 18), then suddenly sexual health also became a potential political challenge to other value systems that might be seen as obstacles with respect to the right to (sexual) health. This has become even more acute in the SDG era and, as we will see, informs various forms of tensions between the State and the individual, between freedom and responsibility, and between a sustainable future or the failure to correct sexual health challenges in time.

Sexual rights

The focus on sexual rights is perhaps the most striking difference between the PAHO 2000 document and the 1987 and 1975 documents. This direct link between sexual health and sexual rights leads to the PAHO adopting eleven sexual rights that in turn had been issued by the WAS, once again also showing how one group of experts, sexologists, has had an enormous influence upon the formation of the concept sexual health. The eleven sexual rights that the PAHO adopted were

> 1. The right to sexual freedom. 2. The right to sexual autonomy, sexual integrity, and safety of the sexual body. 3. The right to sexual privacy. 4. The right to sexual equity. 5. The right to sexual pleasure. 6. The right to emotional expression. 7. The right to sexually associate freely. 8. The right to make free and responsible reproductive choices. 9. The right to sexual information based upon scientific inquiry. 10. The right to comprehensive sexuality education. 11. The right to Sexual health care.
>
> (2000)

The PAHO and subsequently the WHO, who co-sponsored this report, can be said to be doing a lot of "productive work" in enshrining these sexual rights and linking them directly to the term "sexual health." The PAHO inscribes sexual rights within a universal framework that transcends local values and norms. Much like the 1975 document, the PAHO document frames sexual health as being anchored in scientific knowledge and recognizes that value systems do influence the concept of sexual health, yet it overrides this by framing these eleven sexual rights within a "universal value system that overrides specific cultural differences" (Giami, 2002).

This, of course, has opened up various forms of controversies, not unlike the many controversies that are found in the tension between universal human rights, on the one hand, and, on the other, national and local rights and laws. In terms of sexual health and sexual rights, some of the controversies have circled around gender equality, LGBTQI rights, HIV testing anonymity, HIV criminalization, and rights to bodily autonomy expressed through marriage laws (Hawkes & Buse, 2015; Lottes, 2013; Nowicka, 2011). By introducing the concept of sexual rights, the PAHO document also opened up several tension-filled spaces in terms of ensuring, on the one hand, sexual freedom and, on the other, sexual responsibility.

The introduction of sexual rights also seems to beg the question of what role the state should have in this, as well as the obligations that the introduction of such rights would entail. What are the obligations of the state through a set of sexual rights, and, conversely, what obligations are laid on the individual in following up these rights? We will get to these questions later when we will analyze a set of sexual health strategies and action plans made in the aftermath of the SDGs, but suffice it to say that the introduction of rights and responsibilities in the PAHO document has become a pillar within sexual health strategies.

Dual responsibility

While rights were a novel and important introduction to the sexual health framework, the focus on responsibility as highlighted in the PAHO Action Plan was also something new. While sexual responsibility had always been an issue and more often than not been seen through highly moralizing terms within the broader framework of sex, sexuality, and health, what was new in the PAHO plan was the extent to which responsibility was framed as a pillar of sexual health. The Action Plan states that

> Responsible sexual behavior is expressed at the individual, interpersonal and community levels. It is characterized by autonomy, mutuality, honesty, respectfulness, consent, protection, the pursuit of pleasure, and wellness. The person exhibiting responsible sexual behavior does not intend to cause harm and refrains from exploitation, harassment, manipulation, and discrimination. A community promotes responsible sexual behaviors by providing the knowledge, resources, and rights individuals need to engage in these practices.
>
> (Pan American Health Organization, 2000, p. 8)

What strikes us as interesting and important in the previous quote is the clear tone of a dual responsibility, one which is laid at the feet the individual but also the level of the community or the state. Sexual responsibility becomes *everybody's* responsibility. In very clear terms, however, the PAHO definition of sexual responsibility obligates individuals and communities to engage in practices that are responsible; thus, the definition "establishes moral criteria for behavior, which is to preserve and develop health and well-being" (Giami, 2002, p. 20).

Of further interest for us here is how this definition has also laid the foundation for a framework of sexual health which established an understanding that it was individual behavior more than medical interventions that produced and changed sexual health. It should be mentioned here, as we will show later on, that while responsible behavior within the domain of sexual health has dominated many action plans and strategies, we have to state that more and more of this kind of responsible behavior is predicated upon a *specific form of responsible behavior*. More and more, the notion of responsible sexual behavior has become linked to the use of evidence-based information to make rational and risk-calculating sexual health decisions: making sure that one chooses the biomedical intervention that is best suited for the individual (a market logic seen in birth control for women, wherein the choice of the pill and a host of other options comes into play. However, with more and more options also within the field of HIV prevention, the same kind of marketization of sexual health holds sway as well).[1] We will return to some of these dynamics later on, but concerning the development of the term "sexual health," the focus on personal responsibility also becomes key through the framework of the SDGs, as the responsibility to ensure a sustainable sexual health future also creates frictions and tensions between the overarching SDG framework, the national level of sexual health strategies, and the personal wishes and desires of the individuals who are also to conduct themselves in such a manner as to achieve the SDGs related to sexual health.

Sexual health as a public health issue

The last document we will look at to get a firmer grip on the development of the concept of sexual health as it has figured in the WHO and within the UN's many frameworks comes from the US surgeon general's *Call to Action to Promote Sexual Health and Responsible Sexual Behavior*, which was published in 2001 (Satcher, 2001). The rationale for including this Action Plan is that while it was produced for the US, its impact and influence upon subsequent sexual health strategies outside the US and within the WHO and UN system have been strongly linked by many scholars in the field (Edwards & Coleman, 2004; Giami, 2002; Sandfort & Ehrhardt, 2004). Another point of interest is that one of the key persons outside of the US government who was part of the production of the surgeon general's call to action was Eli Coleman, who was the WAS president at the time and had played a major role in writing and editing the PAHO/WHO Action Plan in 2000 (Giami, 2002, p. 22). The 2001 US document builds on the prior documents we have seen but has a clear identity that is firmly anchored in addressing sexual health as a public health issue rather than as an object solely bound to the individual and the individual's rights and needs, as seen earlier. Furthermore, the surgeon general's call for action clearly highlights responsibility and subsequently also risks. The public health perspective was absent in the 1975 document and not dealt with in the 1987 WHO document, and in the 2000 PAHO document, it was noted but in abstract terms. In the 2001 US document, the public health aspects of sexual health are truly highlighted and come to the fore alongside responsibility and risks.

The opening paragraph states:

> I am introducing the Surgeon General's Call to Action to Promote Sexual Health and Responsible Sexual Behavior because we, as a nation, must address the significant public health challenges regarding the sexual health of our citizens. In recognition of these challenges, promoting responsible sexual behavior is included among the Surgeon General's Public Health Priorities.
>
> (Satcher, 2001, p. i)

US Surgeon General David Satcher rhetorically addresses the entire United States and directly links sexual health to public health challenges and, through recourse to "we, as a nation," creates a linguistic injunction to address these issues through responsible sexual health. Satcher goes on to list eight challenges to public health which are connected to sexual health, and, of these eight, four are related to the HIV/AIDS epidemic (Satcher, 2001, p. ii). The introduction to the document finishes off by stating that

> Each of these problems carries with it the potential for lifelong consequences – for individuals, families, communities, and the nation as a whole. As is the case with so many public health problems, there are serious disparities among the populations affected. The economically disadvantaged, racial, and ethnic minorities, persons with different sexual identities, disabled persons, and adolescents often bear the heaviest burden. Yet it is important to recognize that persons of all ages and backgrounds are at risk and should have access to the knowledge and services necessary for optimal sexual health. . . . It is also important to recognize the responsibilities that individuals and communities have in protecting sexual health. The responsibility of well-informed adults as educators and role models for their children cannot be overstated.
>
> (Satcher, 2001, p. ii)

The concluding remarks which are made are telling in that rather than focusing on rights or the universality of sexual health, as we have seen before, the surgeon general notes that while there are disparities within sexual health problems, potentially everyone is at risk for these problems, and it is thus also everyone's responsibility to protect national and individual sexual health. Satcher's statement here seems to point to the symbiotic relationship between the state and the individual. The health of the body politic is seen as intrinsically linked to the personal body of the individual. Risk is also omnipresent and thus needs to be mitigated communally, even though disparities are acknowledged. The biopolitical veneer of this statement should not go unnoticed here. Sexual health is indeed a space wherein the health of the individual and that of the state come in contact in such as way that a biopolitical analysis is well suited to shed light upon the many paradoxes and tensions within such policies and governmental rule.

Inscribing sexual health in the logic of biopolitics

Mutual responsibility between individual and collective as well as the balance between freedom and responsibility is, as we will see in the SDG framework, still a predominant way of framing sexual health. Indeed, some of the arguments in this book are that the individual's freedom, choice, and cultural and religious values often clash with the collective or the state's notion of evidence, norms, and values (both economically and morally). Sexual health as a form of biopolitical space of concern for health authorities can be understood if we use Foucault's link between sex and governance: sex is key in how it allows for biopolitical interventions at both the individual level and at the population level; it fuses the disciplinary power which targets the individual body and the regulatory power aimed at the population level:

> This is the background that enables us to understand the importance assumed by sex as a political issue. It was at the pivot of the two axes along which developed the entire political technology of life. On the one hand, it was tied to the disciplines of the body: the harnessing, intensification, and distribution of forces, the adjustment, and economy of energies. On the other hand, it was applied to the regulation of populations, through all the far-reaching effects of its activity. It fitted in both categories at once, giving rise to infinitesimal surveillances, permanent controls, extremely meticulous orderings of space, indeterminate medical or psychological examinations, to an entire micro-power concerned with the body. But it gave rise as well to comprehensive measures, statistical assessments, and interventions aimed at the entire social body or groups taken as a whole. Sex was a means of access both to the life of the body and the life of the species. It was employed as a standard for the disciplines and as a basis for regulations.
>
> (Foucault, 1990, pp. 145–146)

The term "sexual health," as we have laid its modern history out in the previous follows in line with this sort of logic, we argue. In all of the documents we have analyzed, and in particular the US surgeon general's, the emphasis on the public health aspect of sexual health inscribes itself within the focus that Foucault here mentions. It is, however, interesting to see how the changes from 1975 through to the surgeon general's call to action increasingly, in fact, take on a more and more public health approach, an approach which targets the entire social body through risk rhetoric while at the same time also instilling rights and responsibilities which both discipline and regulate individuals and the body politic in general.

There is also another way in which the surgeon general's document inscribes itself into the logic of biopolitics. Allow us to link the following statement from the 2001 Action Plan to a later quote from Foucault. The US surgeon general's quote reads as follows:

> In the present case, public health responds to the problem – sexually transmitted diseases, unintended pregnancies, and sexual violence – by asking what

is known about its distribution and rates, what factors can be modified, if those modifications are acceptable to the community, and if they are likely to address the problem.

(Satcher, 2001)

Before turning to Foucault, we should briefly state that the quote from the surgeon general's call associates problems with sexual health with those that arise from sexual activity proper; less is said about rights, identity, or freedom as envisioned by prior calls for action. Going back to Foucault, it is almost uncanny how the surgeon general's call in this case echoes some of the points that Foucault has made on the rise of biopolitics and how it relies on just the kind of approaches that the call to action here mentions.

Foucault notes that biopolitics, as it emerged in the 18th century, relied more and more on a new type of power, one in which statistics and various demographic rates – birth rates, death rates, fertility rates, and so on – were seen as instrumental to how society was governed (Foucault, 2003, p. 243). It is clear that the US surgeon general's call to action relies precisely on the biopolitical instruments that Foucault highlighted as the new way of conducting government; Satcher's call is one which relies on surveillance data such as epidemiological metrics of prevalence, incident rates, mortality rates, and the spatialization of these through the wording of "asking what is known about its distribution and rates." Biomedical surveillance is a much clearer part of Satcher's call than in the other definitions that we have looked at. Furthermore, risk enters into this call for action much more than in the other documents, and when combined with the notion of responsible sexual behavior, the rhetoric of surveillance, vigilance, and preemption seems to dominate the US surgeon general's call to action. For instance, the document goes on to note that

Sexual responsibility should be understood in its broadest sense. While personal responsibility is crucial to any individual's health status, communities also have important responsibilities. Individual responsibility includes understanding and awareness of one's sexuality and sexual development; respect for oneself and one's partner; avoidance of physical or emotional harm to either oneself or one's partner; ensuring that pregnancy occurs only when welcomed, and recognition and tolerance of the diversity of sexual values within many communities. Community responsibility includes an assurance that its members have: access to developmentally and culturally appropriate sexuality education, as well as sexual and reproductive health care and counseling; the latitude to make appropriate sexual and reproductive choices; respect for diversity; and freedom from stigmatization and violence based on gender, race, ethnicity, religion, or sexual orientation.

(Satcher, 2001, p. 1)

In formulating this kind of frame for understanding responsible sexual behavior, the report simultaneously states that everybody is responsible for conducting themselves following what is now looking more and more like a normative injunction for sexual behavior. And if we now connect this with the prior quote, which also stated that everyone is potentially at risk for various sexual health problems, risk and responsibility, rhetorically at least, are projected onto everyone and at all levels: individual, communal, and state. In much the same way, this is how the SDG framework also operates; sustainable development is a promise made by a global "we," yet it is up to various local "we" actors to make good on this promise (Engebretsen et al., 2016). At the same time, sustainable development, much like sexual health in the frame offered here, becomes everybody's business, since everybody, at least theoretically, is both at risk and has responsibility for this risk.

Act responsibly – abstinence

The surgeon general's call to action differs not only in the strong tone of responsibility and risk that it uses, but it is also different in that it, contrary to the PAHO and the 1975 document, focuses much less on well-being and the free and responsible expression of sexual ability and much more on understanding risks, acting responsibly, and even abstaining from sex when it is appropriate to do so (Giami, 2002, p. 23). For instance, the PAHO document only mentions abstinence in the appendix, and here it is only meant to be targeted at teenagers (Pan American Health Organization, 2000, p. 41). The theme of abstinence in the surgeon general's call, on the other hand, is much more prominent and is directly linked to the notion of responsibility and risk. The word "abstinence" or "abstain" appears ten times in the surgeon general's call to action, such as in

> Sexual health is not limited to the absence of disease or dysfunction, nor is its importance confined to just the reproductive years. It includes the ability to understand and weigh the risks, responsibilities, outcomes, and impacts of sexual actions and to practice abstinence when appropriate.
>
> (Satcher, 2001, p. 1)

Here, abstinence is part of an ongoing self-monitoring of sexual behavior which every one of us is expected to engage in.

Sexual responsibility includes, therefore, an ongoing disciplining of the self, which, in the surgeon general's call, is predicated less upon the freedom *to* do something, and more on freedom *from* something, which in turn is manifested through self-monitoring and discipline. Risk and responsibility become in this framework driving factors in fostering or rather disciplining healthy sexuality and sexual health both nationally and individually.

> Sexual responsibility is, thus, an individual value and an ideal behavior, supported by a community. The key concept of sexual responsibility is not based on the idea of free involvement in sexual activity but on the ability to make appropriate choices.
>
> (Giami, 2002, p. 23)

While risk and responsibility seem to be omnipresent factors in the fostering of a nationwide healthy sexuality, the surgeon general, as we have seen, does acknowledge that disparities in sexual health are present.

Support and encouragement of people living with HIV

When it comes to the case of HIV, the surgeon general's document singles out people living with HIV (PLHIV) as an "outgroup" which needs to "co-operate" with "us," that is, people who are not living with HIV:

> I would like to add a few words for the many thousands of persons living with HIV/AIDS in this country. We realize that you are not the enemy; that the enemy in this epidemic is the virus, not those who are infected with it. You need our support and encouragement. At the same time, it is also important that you realize you have an opportunity to partner with us in stemming the spread of this illness; to be responsible in your own behavior, and to help others become aware of the need for responsible behavior in their sexual lives. Working together, we can make a difference.
>
> (Satcher, 2001, p. ii)

The quote clearly shows that while the US government, through the surgeon general, "realize that" people living with HIV are not the enemy, they are singled out as an "outgroup" who both need support and encouragement. This in and of itself is not problematic; the issue is rather the rhetoric of "realizing" that one has the opportunity to "partner" up with an "us," which in combination can stem the tide of the HIV/AIDS epidemic through taking on a double burden of responsibility, taking both responsibility for one's sexual behavior as well as that of others by "helping others become aware of the need for responsible behavior in their sexual lives." In the same quote, responsibility is shifted onto PLHIV in such a manner that they are to both conduct themselves according to responsible sexual behavior norms and lead by example and help others become aware of their responsibility and risks.

As we shall see later, this sort of rhetoric has become enshrined in various HIV prevention campaigns wherein HIV prevention and sexual health responsibility have shifted onto more and more individualized tropes in which PLHIV are seen to become responsible for their behavior but also the behavior of others (Sandset, 2019). The notion that it is everyone's responsibility to secure nationwide sexual health seems also to rest on implicit rhetoric wherein certain people are made *more* responsible. This has clear parallels to some of the tropes that we will see in how sustainable development is put in relation to sexual health and sexuality, in particular when it comes to birth control issues and HIV prevention. To paraphrase the quote from *Animal Farm* by George Orwell, "all animals are equal, but some animals are *more* equal than others" (Orwell & Heath, 2003), we could perhaps state that "all individuals are responsible, but some are more responsible than others" for, in this case, HIV prevention. The argument that we are making here is that the rhetorical work that the surgeon general does is just that: there is a doubling of responsibility laid at the feet of PLHIV to be both responsible for their sexual health and that of others.

Concluding remarks

In the 21st century, sex has become an explicit concern of individuals, states, doctors, human rights activists, researchers, and policymakers. It is therefore important to critically investigate how sexual health now figures in the largest public health implementation the world has ever seen, that is, the rollout of the SDGs on a global scale. In this chapter, we tried to give a historical account of the various forms and definitions that the term "sexual health" has taken throughout the years, and by doing so, we hope to have also added to a more nuanced understanding of the term. It is clear that sexual health as a term within the lexicon of public health has changed and that these changes have clear historical and material resonances, such as the introduction of the contraceptive pill, the women's rights movement, LGBTQI rights, and the HIV epidemic. It is also clear that this shifting semiotic meaning throughout the years has led to a certain semiotic polysemy, the nature of which has led to the term to acquiring a vast set of meanings associated with it. This will be important later on in this book, as the polysemy of the term also allows it to operate in such a way that it can be used in many different policy framings. Sustainability, which came to influence sexual health thinking later, might not have had a strong influence on the term in the formative years when it was floated in the WHO vocabulary, yet in later years, sustainability thinking has come to be important for thinking about sexual health. As we soon shall see, this has led to different framings of responsibility, rights, and manners of intervening in the intimate lives of people.

Note

1 Case in point regarding the multiple choices that women have would be Planned Parenthood, whose website on birth control options for women lists a total of eighteen options, all of them laid out with the name of the method, how accurate it is, how it is to be practiced and how effective it is in preventing unplanned pregnancies. For the webpage, see www.plannedparenthood.org/learn/birth-control. In the case of HIV prevention, we have seen a somewhat similar marketization. Here we can mention condoms, pre-exposure prophylaxis (PrEP), post-exposure prophylaxis PEP, and, for people who are living with HIV, there's anti-retroviral treatment (ARV), which leads to untransmittable viral load numbers, thus constituting no risk of onwards transmission. There are also long-acting injectables, which will be available in the not-so-distant future. If we also include practices that have emerged within men who have sex with men (MSM) communities such as negotiated safety, then the total amount of HIV prevention options for the individual amounts to eight.

References

Department of Health, England. (2013). *A framework for sexual health improvement in England.* https://assets.publishing.service.gov.uk/government/uploads/system/ uploads/attachment_data/file/142592/9287-2900714-TSO-SexualHealthPolicyNW_ ACCESSIBLE.pdf

Edwards, W. M., & Coleman, E. (2004). Defining sexual health: A descriptive overview. *Archives of Sexual Behavior, 33*(3), 189–195.

Engebretsen, E., Heggen, K., Das, S., Farmer, P., & Ottersen, O. P. (2016). Paradoxes of sustainability with consequences for health. *The Lancet Global Health, 4*(4), e225–e226.

Epstein, S., & Mamo, L. (2017). The proliferation of sexual health: Diverse social problems and the legitimation of sexuality. *Social Science & Medicine, 188*, 176–190.

Foucault, M. (1990). *The history of sexuality: An introduction* (R. Hurley, trans., vol. I.). Vintage.

Foucault, M. (2003). *"Society Must Be Defended": Lectures at the Collège de France, 1975–1976* (vol. 1). Macmillan.

Giami, A. (2002). Sexual health: The emergence, development, and diversity of a concept. *Annual Review of Sex Research, 13*(1), 1–35.

Giami, A., & Perrey, C. (2012). Transformations in the medicalization of sex: HIV prevention between discipline and biopolitics. *Journal of Sex Research, 49*(4), 353–361.

Hawkes, S., & Buse, K. (2015). Sights set on sexual rights in global culture wars: Implications for health. *The Lancet Global Health Blog, 21.*

Lottes, I. L. (2000). New perspectives on sexual health. *New Views on Sexual Health: The Case of Finland*, 7–29.

Lottes, I. L. (2013). Sexual rights: Meanings, controversies, and sexual health promotion. *Journal of Sex Research, 50*(3–4), 367–391.

Mann, J. M., Gostin, L., Gruskin, S., Brennan, T., Lazzarini, Z., & Fineberg, H. V. (1994). Health and human rights. *Health and Human Rights*, 6–23.

Ministry of Health and Care Services Norway. (2017). *Snakk om det! Strategi for seksuell helse 2017–2022.* https://www.regjeringen.no/contentassets/284e09615fd04338a817e1 160f4b10a7/strategi_seksuell_helse.pdf

Nowicka, W. (2011). Sexual and reproductive rights and the human rights agenda: Controversial and contested. *Reproductive Health Matters, 19*(38), 119–128.

Orwell, G., & Heath, A. (2003). *Animal farm and 1984.* Houghton Mifflin Harcourt.

Pan American Health Organization. (2000). *Promotion of sexual health: Recommendations for action.* Regional Office of the World Health Organization, PAHO.

Public Health England. (2015). *Health promotion for sexual and reproductive health and HIV.* https://assets.publishing.service.gov.uk/government/uploads/system/uploads/attachment_data/file/488090/SRHandHIVStrategicPlan_211215.pdf

Sandfort, T. G., & Ehrhardt, A. A. (2004). Sexual health: A useful public health paradigm or a moral imperative? *Archives of Sexual Behavior, 33*(3), 181–187.

Sandset, T. (2019). "HIV both starts and stops with me": Configuring the neoliberal sexual actor in HIV prevention. *Sexuality & Culture*, 1–17.

Satcher, D. (2001). The surgeon general's call to action to promote sexual health and responsible sexual behavior. *American Journal of Health Education, 32*(6), 356–368.

UNAIDS. (2019). *Global AIDS monitoring 2019: Indicators for the monitoring of the 2016 political declaration on ending AIDS 208.* https://indicatorregistry.unaids.org/sites/default/files/2019-global-aids-monitoring_en_0.pdf

WHO. (1975). *Education and treatment in human sexuality: The training of health professionals, report of a WHO meeting [held in Geneva from 6 to 12 February 1974].* WHO.

WHO. (1987). *Concepts of sexual health: Report of a working group*. Regional Office for Europe, WHO.

WHO. (2002). *Defining sexual health: Report of a technical consultation on sexual health*. WHO.

WHO. (2016). *Action plan for sexual and reproductive health: Towards achieving the 2030 agenda for sustainable development in Europe – leaving no one behind*. WHO.

4 The global promise to "end AIDS"

A double-duty paradox or genuine solidarity?

Introduction

When the UN and its member states signed the SDGs in 2015, the Agenda 2030 document stated that governments, the public and private sectors, and non-governmental organizations were expected to form a "collaborative partnership" in order to realize the plan, which pledges "no one will be left behind" on the road to a sustainable future. Of the seventeen goals, one (SDG3) is specifically dedicated to health, while several others address the environmental, political, social, and economic determinants of health and well-being. Target 3.3 states, "by 2030, end the epidemics of AIDS, tuberculosis" (United Nations, 2015). To end AIDS, as well as reaching the other SDG goals, a total of 169 targets are found within the Agenda 2030 document, as well as a staggering 244 indicators. We argue in this chapter that

> although monitoring the SDGs is undoubtedly important, we believe that the indicators for monitoring the achievement of the goals must be accompanied by critical attention to ambiguities of accountability inherent in the Agenda itself.
>
> (Engebretsen et al., 2017, p. 365)

in particular, when it comes to the notion of ending AIDS by 2030. Agenda 2030 "is making big promises, such as "we are determined to end poverty and hunger, in all their forms." At the same time, the Agenda distinguishes between the "we" making the promise and the "we" that is responsible for keeping it: "we have mapped the road to sustainable development; it will be for all of us to ensure that the journey is successful" (Engebretsen et al., 2017, p. 365). This creates an unresolved tension in the agenda between the global "we" making the promise and the *we* that must be loyal to the promises of the agenda. In this sense, the SDGs are trapped within a similar paradox of authority that Derrida identifies through his reading of the American Declaration of Independence: in order to command authority, the SDGs must state an opinion that is already there; this must represent the "will of the people." However, at the same time, the agenda must qualify something new. If it only stated a given fact, it would be redundant. Thus, in a way, the will of the people is always dictated by an authority. Being drafted by Thomas Jefferson and signed by "the Representatives of the United States of America, in General Congress, Assembled in the Name, and by Authority of the good People," the "we" points to an infinite regress of authority. The authentic voice of the declaration – the identity of the "we" who declare – cannot be decided. Only the name of "God" can close the infinite regress of authority: "appealing to the Supreme Judge of the world for the rectitude of our intentions." Derrida argues that because the Declaration is based on being "undecidable between . . . a performative structure and a constitutive structure," "one cannot decide whether independence is stated or produced by this utterance" (Derrida, 1986, p. 49). There is, of course, a difference between the Declaration of Independence and the UNs SDGs. The "future deferral" of "we" that Derrida focuses on is, it seems, different than the SDGs, which are put forth by an already constructed global community, albeit a sometimes fragile and fractured global community. Yet, as we have argued elsewhere, the (sometimes) divided "we" in the SDG agenda makes it difficult to determine whether the SDGs are stated or produced by the Agenda and whether the goals are declared or enforced (Engebretsen et al., 2017).

As we will demonstrate in the following, this dual "we" blurring the distinction between promise and order is particularly visible in the discourse related to the aim of ending AIDS. In 2016, UNAIDS officially adopted the "Political Declaration on HIV and AIDS: On the Fast Track to Accelerating the Fight against HIV and to Ending the AIDS Epidemic by 2030" (UNAIDS, 2015). In the Declaration, the Heads of States pledged to "reaffirm *our* commitment to end the AIDS epidemic by 2030" by accelerating the fight against HIV and ending AIDS (italics added, UNAIDS, 2015). Furthermore, the Declaration identified HIV and AIDS as a global emergency that represents a formidable challenge to the development, progress, and stability of the world and requires a comprehensive global response" (UNAIDS, 2015). Another instance of such a use of a "we" can be found in strategies from PEPFAR, the world's largest donor of HIV funding to low and middle income countries (LMICs), who have also made similar promises. In PEPFAR's *Controlling the Epidemic. Delivering on the Promise of an AIDS-Free Generation*, a promise of ensuring an AIDS-free generation is made, yet, as PEPFAR states, "we cannot do this alone. We need partnerships with organizations; other donor nations, civil society, and multilateral institutions, and we need on-the-ground partners and governments who are vital to controlling the epidemic in their countries" (PEPFAR, 2015, p. 7).

In this chapter, we will scrutinize the paradox of authority inherent in these strategies committed to ending AIDS. Based on a critical and deconstructive reading, we argue that there is a potential double-duty paradox embedded in the global "promise" to end AIDS as it is articulated in all these documents. Paraphrasing Engebretsen et al., we can state that "the end of AIDS is about both committing oneself to a promise and committing others to an obligation, it both *declares* and *enforces* its commitment" (Engebretsen et al., 2017, p. 365). Moreover, we argue that the promise to end AIDS often ends up becoming *an obligation laid at the feet of individuals rather than a form of collective responsibility to change broader structural drivers of the epidemic.* Rather than exonerating *everyone* of their responsibility to end AIDS, the ambiguity of responsibility formed through the recourse of a global "we" might end up *individualizing* and *biomedicalizing* the promise to end AIDS.

In our final analysis, we contend that the double-duty paradox ends up obligating individuals through neoliberal mechanisms predicated upon notions of rational choice, risk calculation, and market choice for HIV treatment and prevention.

Global promises: ending AIDS in the Sustainable Development Goal era

In the preamble to the Agenda 2030 document, we can read that "we are determined to end poverty and hunger, in all their forms and dimensions" (United Nations, 2015, p. 3). Furthermore,

> we are resolved to, between now and 2030, to end poverty and hunger everywhere; to combat inequalities within and amongst countries; to build peaceful, just and inclusive societies; to protect human rights and promote gender equality and the empowerment of women.
>
> (United Nations, 2015, p. 4)

The Agenda also pledges that to

> promote physical and mental health and well-being and to extend life expectancy *for all, we* must achieve universal health coverage and access to quality health care. *No one must be left behind. . . . We will* equally accelerate the pace of progress made in fighting malaria, *HIV/AIDS*, tuberculosis, hepatitis, Ebola and other communicable diseases and epidemics.
>
> (italics added, United Nations, 2015, p. 7)

The SDGs thus formulate a strong "we" who promises and pledges to, amongst other things, end AIDS, and "leave no one behind" while also ensuring that "those that are furthest behind come first" (United Nations, 2015, p. 3).

On the one hand, the SDGs formulates a "we" that pledges to end AIDS, making a promise "on behalf of the peoples we serve" (United Nations, 2015, p. 3). However, on the other hand, "the Agenda distinguishes between the 'we' making the promise and the 'we' that is responsible for keeping it" (Engebretsen et al., 2017, p. 365). After the Agenda has proclaimed its vision and made its pledges, it goes on to state that

> As *we* embark on this great collective journey, *we* pledge that no one will be left behind. . . . It is *"we* the peoples" who are embarking today on the road to 2030. *Our* journey will involve Governments as well as parliaments, the United Nations system and other international institutions, local authorities, indigenous peoples, civil society, business, and the private sector, the

scientific and academic community – and all people. . . . *We* have mapped the road to sustainable development; it will be for *all of us* to ensure that the journey is successful and its gains irreversible.

(italics added, United Nations, 2015, p. 12)

The Agenda states that there is a "we" who pledges to reach the SDG goals while at the same time engendering another broader "we." "By mapping the road, the first 'we' has done its deed. It is now up to a new and broader 'we' to "ensure that the journey is successful" (Engebretsen et al., 2017, p. 365). This introduces a double-duty paradox: on the one hand, to end AIDS through the lens of the SDGs becomes a *promise* made by a global "we." Yet, on the other hand, the statement also *obligates* others, as can be discerned through the interpellation of "governments as well as parliaments, the United Nations system and other international institutions, local authorities, indigenous peoples, civil society, business and the private sector, the scientific and academic community – and all people."

In the *Political Declaration on HIV and AIDS: On the Fast Track to Accelerating the Fight against HIV and to Ending the AIDS Epidemic by 2030* signed by the UN General Assembly on 8 June 2016, we can find a similar paradox. In the declaration,

We, Heads of State and Government and representatives of States and Governments assembled at the United Nations from 8 to 10 June 2016, reaffirm *our* commitment to end the AIDS epidemic by 2030 as *our* legacy to present and future generations . . . to accelerate and scale up the fight against HIV and end AIDS.

(UNAIDS, 2015, p. 1)

The declaration goes on to state that "we pledge to intensify efforts towards the goal of comprehensive prevention, treatment, care and support programmes" (UNAIDS, 2015, p. 1). The undecidability between the performative and constitutive aspect of the declaration is here visible in the choice of words. On the one hand, the text *declares* a "goal," but, on the other hand, this declaration is a reaffirmation of an already existing "commitment" and "legacy" which the text only "accelerates" or "scales up." Hence, the goal is both produced and reaffirmed through the text. This rhetorical move makes it possible to emphasize the declaration as a visionary promise and as a shared responsibility at the same time. Once again, the promise to end AIDS is formulated through a "we," a global "we" which pledges to end AIDS within 2030. Yet again, the interpellation of a broader "we" can be discerned through sections such as the following:

Encourage *all regions* to work with regional and subregional organizations, people living with, at risk of and affected by HIV, relevant United Nations system organizations, the private sector and other relevant stakeholders towards the achievement of the following targets by 2020, as modelled in the fast-track approach to ending the AIDS epidemic by 2030, and, in this regard, call for strengthened global solidarity and *shared responsibility*.

> (italics added, UNAIDS, 2015, p. 23)

The global promise made by the first "we" is supplemented by an emphasis on *all* relevant stakeholders, and that responsibility is *shared*. The promise is also an obligation. Hence, the mechanisms of accountability are hard to discern with the risk of making the end of AIDS "everyone's business but no-one's major responsibility" (Engebretsen et al., 2017, p. 365). Engebretsen et al. have rightly pointed out that

> should we even come close to achieving the SDGs, we must be able to hold specific agents to account. The responsibility for achieving the goals cannot be entrusted to an unidentifiable and all-encompassing "we." If everyone is accountable in theory, no one is accountable in practice.
>
> (2017, p. 365)

Pledges to end AIDS by recourse to a "we" are also found within key UNAIDS reports and rhetoric. We can also here see the contours of a double-duty paradox emerging. Take, for example, the recent UNAIDS report *Miles to Go* (UNAIDS, 2018). In the foreword by former Executive Director Michel Sidibé, we can read the following:

> AIDS is not over, but it can be. At the halfway point to the 2020 targets, *we must recommit* ourselves to achieve them. The successes in HIV treatment show what can be done when *we* put our minds to it. People living with HIV are leading longer, healthier lives. But *we* still have miles to go. *We have promises to keep.*
>
> (italics added, UNAIDS, 2018, p. 7)

With direct reference to the promise to end AIDS, Sidibé formulates a promise made by a primary "we." Yet it is not altogether clear *who* this "we" is. Another citation from the same report might illuminate this argument further. The report goes on to state that

> As we reflect on our progress, some satisfaction is warranted. But on balance, the world is slipping off track. The promises made to society's most vulnerable individuals are not being kept. There are miles to go on the journey to end the AIDS epidemic. Time is running out.
>
> (UNAIDS, 2018, p. 9)

Once again, there is a primary "we" that has made some progress, yet the promises made to "society's most vulnerable" are not being kept. The question of who is *not keeping their word* is harder to discern. Even though data is presented on various metrics and issues within the global HIV effort in *Miles to Go*, responsibility for keeping the promise of ending AIDS within 2030 is harder to place. All of the previous reports, strategies, and statements say more about who should pledge to end AIDS and how to end AIDS but little about who *is not* keeping their promise.

Another instance of a global or plural "we" which has emerged within the SDG era is to be found within PEPFAR rhetoric (The President's Emergency Plan For AIDS Relief). Take, for instance, this quote from PEPFAR's *Strategy for Accelerating HIV/AIDS Epidemic Control*:

> We are at a historic moment in the global HIV/AIDS response. For the first time in modern history, we have the opportunity to change the very course of the HIV pandemic, by actually controlling it without a vaccine or a cure. For the first time, the end of the epidemic as a public health threat is in sight.[1]

Who this "we" is might not be as clear-cut, since Tillerson might be referring to PEPFAR as an entity, or he might be referring to a global audience. However, PEPFAR's statement that there is a historic opportunity to end AIDS shared by this "we" is quickly followed by an obligation or at least a form of imploring another set of actors to do *their part*. Directly, PEPFAR states that

> we cannot do this alone. All partners – from governments, the private sector, philanthropy, multilateral institutions, civil society, the faith community, and others – must step up their efforts if we, as a global community, are to control, and ultimately end, this pandemic.[2]

Clearly then, the opportunity and promise to end AIDS are also an obligation made of others. Everyone must step up their efforts if we are to end AIDS.

This, however, might result in a glossing over of potential conflict and power asymmetries in both the implementation of the SDGs and the broader end of AIDS implementation as it figures in UNAIDS reports and documents (Engebretsen et al., 2016, 2017). In a similar vein, Kenworthy et al. have asked us to contemplate what it means to "end AIDS"; that is, what

> does the End of AIDS signify, and for whom? Who stands to benefit from a triumphalism that few believe but many endorse? And most importantly, what kinds of AIDS response does this discourse promote, and what forms of knowledge is it rooted in?
>
> (Kenworthy et al., 2018b, p. 962)

With its consensus-oriented rhetoric and its double-duty paradox, the promise to end AIDS might undermine itself first by glossing over of potential conflicts within the SDGs and the UNAIDS 90–90–90 targets. Second, it might displace responsibility from communal and broad structural initiatives that would tackle syndemic factors such as mental health; socioeconomic access to treatment and prevention; and structural issues such as stigma, discrimination, and racism onto biomedically mediated personalized and individual obligations to end AIDS.

If in the SDGs and the political declaration to end AIDS there is a primary "we" who has "mapped the road to" both sustainable development as well as the end of the AIDS epidemic within 2030, then the *obligation* to make good on this promise might not be implemented through the same primary "we." Rather we will argue in the following that implementation of efforts to "end AIDS" by 2030 end up *obligating* individuals to engage with biomedical technologies of treatment and prevention. The collective journey to end AIDS, as it is referred to in the SDGs, might have been mapped by a primary and global "we," but, as we shall see, it is often left to the individual to make good on this promise through obligations to adhere to, and engage with, various biomedical technologies of treatment and prevention. A brief look at some prominent and contemporary HIV campaigns in the United States and England can partly substantiate our analysis.

"HIV both starts and stops with me": from a global promise to a personal obligation

The collective "we," which makes a promise to end AIDS, is almost omnipresent within the current drive to end AIDS. Take, for example, New York City's "Ending the Epidemic" strategy[3] and its "Play Sure" campaign.[4] Following the announcement of the mayor of NYC, Bill de Blasio, "Play Sure" was rolled out with a live event wherein de Blasio, as Thomann describes, was standing "in front of a large screen that read 'From Vision to Reality, #EndAIDSNYC2020'" (2018, p. 1001). At the same event, de Blasio said,

> *We* are resolved to end this epidemic. *We* have the tools. *We're* committed to using them. There's no hesitation. There's no delay . . . the time is now to end the epidemic once and for all. It's as simple as that.
>
> (italics added by authors, Thomann, 2018, p. 1001)

Subsequently, the City of New York announced that it would earmark 23 million dollars starting from the fiscal year of 2017 and every subsequent year after that as part of a statewide plan to reduce new HIV infections to below 750 annually by 2020.[5] Also part of this was the introduction of the "Play Sure" health promotion, a social media marketing campaign which included posters on subways and busses as well as a website[6] and YouTube videos.[7] The health promotion focuses on the "take-home message" of "Be Sure, Play Sure, Stay Sure" and uses the headline of "Together we can stop the spread of HIV and other sexually transmitted infections (STIs)."[8] Through the slogan of "Be Sure. Play Sure. Stay Sure," the campaign plays on the notion of staying "sure," that is, mitigating risk and taking action to do so through testing to be sure and the use of condoms and water-based lubrication in order to "play sure." Finally, in order to "stay sure," the individual is encouraged to "use PrEP" or people living with HIV to stay on treatment in order to "stay sure."[9] However, the target or focus of the campaign is highly individualized. Under the heading of "Be Sure," to be "sure" is equated with "knowing *your* HIV status" and to "know *your* STI status." Specifically, to be sure is to get tested either at least annually or, if you are a MSM or transgender person, every three to six months.[10] To play sure is personalized through the usage of condoms and lubrication, and here the ad promotes choice in stating that "find a condom that works best for you."[11] Finally, to "stay sure" is to either go on PrEP or stay on treatment. For people who are living with HIV, the health promotion focuses on the individual through statements such as

> Starting and staying on treatment can keep your viral load undetectable. Treatment keeps you healthy and can eliminate the risk of passing HIV to your sexual partners. HIV care is not just about taking medications. Even if you feel well, see an HIV doctor regularly to learn how to stay healthy.[12]

The focus here is on the individual to stay sure, which in effect is to mitigate an omnipresent risk through testing, treating, and the continual surveillance of both one's risks as well as one's own body.

While we are not offering a critique of access to and use of PrEP, condoms, and ARVs, we want to point out the apparent disjuncture between global promises made in global strategies and the local obligations laid at the feet of people. Our concern is that the double-duty paradox might lead to a neo-liberalization of the end of AIDS, which in turn presupposes a specific subject that can engage with biomedical treatment and prevention technologies.

There is an interesting shift here in responsibility which is connected to the biomedicalization of HIV and going from a global "we" to a singular "I." The ambiguous responsibility created by the double-duty paradox facilitates a individualization of responsibility through the focus on biomedical solutions. By focusing on *individual and biomedical factors of HIV* transmission, the "we" recedes into the background, and what is highlighted are the individual and singular pharmaceutical solutions such as PrEP and ARVs. Yet structural disparities and access to health care are left untouched by the narrative. We can link this better to how some scholars have conceptualized neoliberalism and health care.

Sastry and Dutta note that

> in the context of health and the intersection between a neoliberal actor and a neoliberal society, assumptions about health are oftentimes started from the notion that 1) health is largely an individual and private responsibility, 2) that ill-health is caused by allocative and technical inefficiencies, and 3), that health can be improved through, for example, cost-effective interventions and the increase of market forces in health services so as to increase choice of treatment and care.
>
> (2012, p. 24)

This focus on the individual within the neoliberalization of health and care stands in stark contrast to the "aspirational," communal, and norm-setting agenda of the SDGs (Kanie & Biermann, 2017). In the case of the global HIV effort,

Thomann highlights the links to the rise of the neoliberal sexual actor when he states that

> the neoliberal sexual actor is one who is configured within health promotions as being one who takes personal responsibility for staying "safe" within the context of HIV, who has the ability to draw upon free-market options and one who makes rational choices in line with "best practice medicine."
>
> (2018, p. 1002)

Going back to the "Play Sure" and the English "It Starts with Me" campaign, we can see these aspects coming to the fore. In one of the ads from the "Play Sure" health promotions, we see the image of two men holding each other, with the tag-line "Be HIV sure. One night can change your HIV status. Be safe, be sure. And get tested frequently."[13] Once again, we see the continual focus on the omnipresence of HIV as a risk that needs to be mitigated through continual surveillance of the individual's perceived HIV risk.

If we now recall the telling turn of events in the Agenda 2030 document, wherein there is a primary "we" who has "mapped the road ahead" towards a sustainable future (and in connection to this, the end of AIDS), but it is "now up to all of us to complete the journey," then in the previous, the promise to end AIDS has now become relegated into a "we" that is encouraged to "play sure." "We play sure" can be read as the transfer of the promise to end AIDS from one primary "we" to another, this time men who have sex with men. The danger as we see it is that this *encouragement* to contribute to the end of AIDS will become coercion, the forcing of normative prescriptions in terms of sexual and intimate behavior, and that the promise to end AIDS will become framed in individualized terms, making the communal promise to end AIDS an *individual obligation*.

Much the same focus on the individual can be seen in the "It Starts with Me" campaign. Just like the "Play Sure" ad focuses on the engagement of the subject with PrEP, ART, testing, and condoms, it also configures a specific individual. The main webpage of the "It Starts with Me" campaign shows a slideshow of four men, all of them with the slogan "I'm stopping HIV," followed by a modality for stopping HIV. These modalities are "I'm stopping HIV," followed by: "I take PrEP," "I use condoms," "I test regularly," and "I am on treatment."[14] Much like the "Play Sure" campaign, the underlying rationale for stopping HIV and ending AIDS lies in the engagement that the individual is having with biomedical interventions such as condoms, PrEP, testing, and treatment. Much like the "Play Sure" campaign, we find a reference to a "we" when the site states that "Together we are stopping HIV. Here's how:".[15] After this, the site lists that in order to "stop AIDS," "we all need to look after ourselves" by "testing at least once a year," by "starting treatment as soon as possible," and finally "to protect," which is mediated by either PrEP or treatment.

Once again, we can extend the argument of the double-duty paradox to cover the "It Starts with Me" campaign; the global promise made by UNAIDS and the

SDGs to end AIDS is formulated through a communal effort that calls upon us all to do our part. Yet, paraphrasing Engebretsen et al., we can say that within the SDGs and the UNAIDS strategies, there is a "mapping [of] the road towards [the end of AIDS], [wherein] the first 'we' has done its deed. It is now up to a new and broader 'we' to 'ensure that the journey is successful'" (Engebretsen et al., 2017, p. 365). In the "It Starts with Me" campaign, we both see the individualized responsibility being highlighted as well as how the end of AIDS is now, at the local level, being made the obligation of another set of "we" communities. "We all need to look after ourselves" can be seen as the textual manifestation of this new "we" that is now obligated to make good on the promise to end AIDS. The end of AIDS and the double-duty paradox which we have worked through in the previous might, in turn, lead to two interlocking challenges and concerns which we share with Kenworthy et al.:

> The "End of AIDS" may likely herald – and justify – two notable shifts in HIV policy: first, the tapering of donor support for long-term treatment (especially for the social and health systems that enable it); and second, a pronounced embrace of technical, often short-term, fixes – a "biomedical turn" that has significant impacts on civil society, health systems, and the real futures of the epidemic.
>
> (2018b, p. 962)

The first part of Kenworthy et al.'s concern is particularly problematic if the tapering of donor funding is done through recourse to what are considered "sustainable" and "not sustainable" HIV initiatives (Engebretsen et al., 2016; Yang et al., 2010). A case in point might be the insights on the "conceptual shift" of the very term "sustainability" as laid out by Engebretsen et al. (2016). Arguing that there has been a shift in the conceptual meaning of sustainability, Engebretsen et al. state that sustainable development, and an extension to this, HIV funding as well, has undergone a transformation wherein the concept in its beginning was associated with durability or development which lasts (Engebretsen et al., 2016, p. e225). From this associative meaning, we have seen a change wherein sustainable health efforts now have come more and more to be associated with "'continuous improvement' as well as with 'monitoring' and systems which are 'domestically driven'" (Engebretsen et al., 2016, p. e225). Furthermore, with "the ideal of continuous improvement incorporated in the current concept of sustainability comes new expectations of self-management and self-assistance" (Engebretsen et al., 2016, p. e225). If the end of AIDS seen from a sustainable development perspective can also be said to labor under this same shift in conceptual meaning, then we postulate that

> An important aspect of the conceptual transformations is that the term sustainability has gradually changed from being a goal (durability) to acquiring connotations that serve as a selection criterion for development aid. Using sustainability as a selection criterion risks privileging recipients who have the

capacity to gain control over health and living conditions and exclude others as unworthy needy.

(Engebretsen et al., 2016, p. e225)

This can also be linked to our argument in this paper: while the global promise to end AIDS is often refracted through a communal effort, it nevertheless also ends up obligating a range of local actors, often in ways that seem to highlight individualized obligations based on biomedical solutions to an epidemic, which is highly driven by social inequalities. In the health promotions mentioned previously, broader societal drivers of the epidemic are left out, and no mention of so-called syndemic vectors are mentioned, thus leaving out issues such as poverty, homelessness, and mental health as important factors. The focus in the images is much more directly on the individual, as well as highlighting the role of biomedical interventions while once again leaving aside any syndemic drivers. As such, the "Play Sure" campaign and the "It Starts with me" promotion both focus on the individual and their engagement with biomedical prevention technologies.

Concluding remarks on the double-duty paradox to end AIDS

While we acknowledge that not every health promotion can target all of the different groups affected by or at risk of HIV, we maintain that the omission of structural drivers such as drug use, discrimination either based on homo-/transphobia or racism and psychological stressors such as depression, isolation, and anxiety is problematic. Mimiaga et al. found that men who have multiple risk factors were much more likely to seroconvert compared to those without risk factors (Mimiaga et al., 2015). The notion that HIV risk is randomly distributed amongst men who have sex with men belies the fact that HIV risk is particularly concentrated in the 10 to 20 percent of MSM or transgender women who are caught in intersecting syndemic conditions (Adam et al., 2017; Bruce & Harper, 2011; Chakrapani et al., 2017; Dyer et al., 2012; González-Guarda et al., 2011; Kurtz et al., 2012; Singer et al., 2017). The danger is not the scale-up of health promotions such as these nor the rollout of ART, testing, and PrEP regimes. Rather the problem as we see it is if the promise made to end AIDS in the SDGs and UNAIDS reports ends up with a local obligation which configures a subject only in an individualized and neoliberal fashion, this might risk the end of AIDS becoming a neoliberal project (Weber, 2015, 2017). In turn, this might risk neoliberal ideas about personal responsibility and obligations becoming doxic *themselves*, which might leave aside the focus on the structural drivers of HIV risk. If these campaigns are any indication of the configuration of the individual who is "to end AIDS," then we can expect more health promotions that focus on the neoliberal sexual citizen as one who is a "pre-emptive patient-consumer" who is made responsible not through risk avoidance but rather through the consumption of biomedical interventions (Thomann, 2018, p. 1002). If this is the outcome of the global promise to end AIDS, then the displacement of responsibility onto local communities and individuals might risk leaving people behind. Furthermore, if the double-duty paradox as we have described it previously is correct, then promising to end AIDS from "global centers of calculation" (Latour, 1987) soon becomes someone else's local moral obligation (Cormier McSwiggin, 2017; Persson et al., 2017). The danger is that those that do not have access to these biomedical preventive technologies, who cannot afford them, or who cannot adhere to them for whatever reason, be that transient homelessness, mental health issues, or economic issues wherein income and insurance are unstable, will be "left behind."

This paradox can be articulated through Thurka Sangaramoorthy's provocation on the current drive to "end AIDS" when she asks us to consider the following:

> There is an inherently powerful and complex paradox underlying the science and practice of HIV/AIDS prevention, which is embodied both by the "We All Have AIDS" campaign's focus on collective advocacy mobilized to combat HIV/AIDS around the globe and by the staggeringly disproportionate rates of HIV/AIDS in many places, like Miami. HIV/AIDS prevention makes claims about the universal impact of HIV/AIDS and the ensuing social responsibility that we all have through multimedia campaigns like "We All Have AIDS". At the same time, HIV/AIDS prevention efforts focus on "higher-risk populations" and divide groups of people through the use of categories of social difference – that is, race, ethnicity, sexual orientation.
>
> (2014, p. 5)

Sangaramoorthy's provocation is also useful for us in asking how the SDGs, PEPFAR, and UNAIDS and their target to end AIDS make claims about the universal impact of disease prevention and eradication measures. They make broad pledges through a primary "we" subject that will end AIDS. As such, they focus on collective agency, responsibility, and solidarity through a universal "we." Yet, HIV/AIDS issues, in general, are often refracted through disparities in health care based on structural inequalities. Furthermore, and as will become apparent a bit later in this book, some communities bear the burden of disease more than others, and public health initiatives more often than not base their efforts precisely on efforts that *divide* people more than *unifying* them. Put rather bluntly: in Sangaramoorthy's example, *not everyone has AIDS*. Some people *do carry* this burden more than others. We argue that Sangaramoorthy's argument can be re-framed within the double-duty paradox we offer in the chapter, and through this, there is a danger that while global actors such as PEPFAR, UN, and UNAIDS can pledge to end AIDS, some people are *made obligated to end AIDS more than others*.

In an age wherein PrEP, ART, and the very discourse of HIV treatment and prevention are riding on the coattails of a discourse of "ending AIDS" (Kenworthy et al., 2018a, 2018b), the slogan of "leaving no one behind" (Weber, 2017; WHO, 2016) in the struggle to "end AIDS" by 2030 might be in danger. If the promise to end AIDS made in the name of a global "we" becomes a double-duty paradox wherein the obligation to make good on this promise is laid at the feet of individuals and only through neoliberal ideas of how health is to be governed, then we might end up with a patchwork effort wherein those of us who are the most vulnerable will be "left behind."

Notes

1 PEPFAR. www.state.gov/wp-content/uploads/2019/08/PEPFAR-Strategy-for-Accelerating-HIVAIDS-Epidemic-Control-2017-2020.pdf
2 Ibid.
3 See NYC's EtE Strategy. http://etedashboardny.org/
4 See the "Play Sure" webpage. https://www1.nyc.gov/site/doh/health/health-topics/playsure.page
5 See New York City site for page on the strategy. https://www1.nyc.gov/office-of-the-mayor/news/578-18/de-blasio-administration-historic-low-new-hiv-diagnoses-down-64-percent-since
6 See the NYC Health website for the "Play Sure" promotion. https://www1.nyc.gov/site/doh/health/health-topics/hiv-besure-playsure-staysure.page
7 See YouTube for examples of videos with the search criteria of "Play Sure" and "HIV." www.youtube.com/results?search_query=play+sure+HIV
8 See the Play Sure website. https://www1.nyc.gov/site/doh/health/health-topics/hiv-besure-playsure-staysure.page
9 Ibid.
10 Ibid.
11 Ibid.
12 Ibid.
13 See the ad here. www.thebody.com/article/new-york-citys-new-hiv-awareness-campaign-shows-in
14 See "It Starts with Me." www.startswithme.org.uk/
15 Ibid.

References

Adam, B. D., Hart, T. A., Mohr, J., Coleman, T., & Vernon, J. (2017). HIV-related syndemic pathways and risk subjectivities among gay and bisexual men: A qualitative investigation. *Culture, Health & Sexuality, 19*(11), 1254–1267.

Bruce, D., & Harper, G. W. (2011). Operating without a safety net: Gay male adolescents and emerging adults' experiences of marginalization and migration, and implications for theory of syndemic production of health disparities. *Health Education & Behavior, 38*(4), 367–378.

Chakrapani, V., Newman, P. A., Shunmugam, M., Logie, C. H., & Samuel, M. (2017). Syndemics of depression, alcohol use, and victimisation, and their association with HIV-related sexual risk among men who have sex with men and transgender women in India. *Global Public Health, 12*(2), 250–265.

Cormier McSwiggin, C. (2017). Moral adherence: HIV treatment, undetectability, and stigmatized viral loads among Haitians in South Florida. *Medical Anthropology*, 1–15.

Derrida, J. (1986). Declarations of independence. *New Political Science, 7*(1), 7–15.

Dyer, T. P., Shoptaw, S., Guadamuz, T. E., Plankey, M., Kao, U., Ostrow, D., Chmiel, J. S., Herrick, A., & Stall, R. (2012). Application of syndemic theory to black men who have sex with men in the multicenter AIDS cohort study. *Journal of Urban Health, 89*(4), 697–708.

Engebretsen, E., Heggen, K., Das, S., Farmer, P., & Ottersen, O. P. (2016). Paradoxes of sustainability with consequences for health. *The Lancet Global Health, 4*(4), e225–e226.

Engebretsen, E., Heggen, K., & Ottersen, O. P. (2017). The Sustainable Development Goals: Ambiguities of accountability. *The Lancet, 389*(10067), 365.

González-Guarda, R. M., Florom-Smith, A. L., & Thomas, T. (2011). A syndemic model of substance abuse, intimate partner violence, HIV infection, and mental health among Hispanics. *Public Health Nursing, 28*(4), 366–378.

Kanie, N., & Biermann, F. (2017). *Governing through goals: Sustainable Development Goals as governance innovation.* MIT Press.

Kenworthy, N., Thomann, M., & Parker, R. (2018a). Critical perspectives on the "end of AIDS". *Global Public Health,* 1–3.

Kenworthy, N., Thomann, M., & Parker, R. (2018b). From a global crisis to the "end of AIDS": New epidemics of signification. *Global Public Health, 13*(8), 960–971.

Kurtz, S. P., Buttram, M. E., Surratt, H. L., & Stall, R. D. (2012). Resilience, syndemic factors, and serosorting behaviors among HIV-positive and HIV-negative substance-using MSM. *AIDS Education and Prevention, 24*(3), 193–205.

Latour, B. (1987). *Science in action: How to follow scientists and engineers through society.* Harvard University Press.

Mimiaga, M. J., O'Cleirigh, C., Biello, K. B., Robertson, A. M., Safren, S. A., Coates, T. J., Koblin, B. A., Chesney, M. A., Donnell, D. J., & Stall, R. D. (2015). The effect of psychosocial syndemic production on 4-year HIV incidence and risk behavior in a large cohort of sexually active men who have sex with men. *Journal of Acquired Immune Deficiency Syndromes (1999), 68*(3), 329.

PEPFAR (2015). *Controlling the epidemic. delivering on the promise of an AIDS-free generation.*

Persson, A., Newman, C. E., & Ellard, J. (2017). Breaking binaries? Biomedicine and serostatus borderlands among couples with mixed HIV status. *Medical Anthropology, 36*(8), 699–713.

Sangaramoorthy, T. (2014). *Treating AIDS: Politics of difference, paradox of prevention.* Rutgers University Press.

Sastry, S., & Dutta, M. J. (2012). Public health, global surveillance, and the "emerging disease" worldview: A postcolonial appraisal of PEPFAR. *Health Communication, 27*(6), 519–532.

Singer, M., Bulled, N., Ostrach, B., & Mendenhall, E. (2017). Syndemics and the biosocial conception of health. *The Lancet, 389*(10072), 941–950.

Thomann, M. (2018). "On December 1, 2015, sex changes. Forever": Pre-exposure prophylaxis and the pharmaceuticalisation of the neoliberal sexual subject. *Global Public Health,* 1–10.

UNAIDS. (2015). *UNAIDS 2016–2021 strategy: on the fast-track to end AIDS.* UNAIDS.

UNAIDS. (2018). *Miles to go – closing gaps, breaking barriers, righting injustices.* Document 268. UNAIDS.United Nations. (2015). *Transforming our world: The 2030 agenda for sustainable development.* Resolution adopted by the General Assembly on 25: 70/1. Seventieth United Nations General Assembly.

Weber, H. (2015). Reproducing inequalities through development: The MDGs and the politics of method. *Globalizations, 12*(4), 660–676.

Weber, H. (2017). Politics of "leaving no one behind": Contesting the 2030 Sustainable Development Goals agenda. *Globalizations, 14*(3), 399–414.

WHO. (2016). *Action plan for sexual and reproductive health: Towards achieving the 2030 agenda for sustainable development in Europe – leaving no one behind.* WHO.

Yang, A., Farmer, P. E., & McGahan, A. M. (2010). "Sustainability" in global health. *Global Public Health, 5*(2), 129–135.

5 Problematizing "sexual health"

Introduction

The concept of sexual health has come to point to several different key elements within the SDGs such as SDG number 3.3 which is "By 2030, end the epidemics of AIDS, tuberculosis, malaria and neglected tropical diseases and combat hepatitis, water-borne diseases, and other communicable diseases" (UN, 2015). Another of the SDGs which is indexed through the contemporary usage of sexual health are SDG goals 3.1 and 3.7, wherein the former reads, "By 2030, reduce the global maternal mortality ratio to less than 70 per 100,000 births" and the latter reads, "By 2030, ensure universal access to sexual and reproductive health-care services, including for family planning, information and education, and the integration of reproductive health into national strategies and programmes" (UN, 2015). Finally, the term "sexual health" is often connected to SDG 5.3, "Eliminate all harmful practices, such as child, early and forced marriage and female genital mutilation" (UN, 2015) and 5.6, which reads "Ensure universal access to sexual and reproductive health and reproductive rights as agreed following the Programme of Action of the International Conference on Population and Development and the Beijing Platform for Action and the outcome documents of their review conferences" (UN, 2015). However, this way of linking the concept of sexual health to such a diverse set of goals, targets, and indicators can only have come about if the concept of sexual health has some form of "polysemy and mutability" of its semantic meaning (Epstein & Mamo, 2017, p. 178). As we have shown earlier in this book, the very concept of sexual health has developed and evolved in relationship to diverse social and political contexts such as the rise of the LGBTQ rights movement, the introduction of the contraceptive pill (popularized as "the pill" many places), the rise of HIV/AIDS as a global epidemic, and the emergence of sexology as a professional expert group and academic endeavor. While these developments are part and parcel of the multitude of reasons sexual health has come to be so polysemic and mutable, this chapter will mainly focus on how this very polysemy and mutability manage to make sexual health a concept which allows governments to use it in such a fashion that it comes to be able to address diverse social issues all in the name of sexual health and the aftermath of the SDGs, the concept of sustainability.

This chapter will seek to uncover some of the silences and omitted areas of sexual health and human sexuality, such as pleasure and desire, two key terms within human sexuality which nevertheless are all but absent in public policy discourse. The argument will be made that many national strategies that deal with sexual health in the SDG era proclaim they are holistic and human-centered, yet desire and pleasure as part of human sexuality and well-being are glossed over and entirely omitted. Indeed, the argument can be made that sexual health as an object of health governance seems to foreclose any reading of pleasure as part of health and human sexuality. The question that remains, then, is: How sustainable is it to produce multiple strategies, reports, and commentaries on sexual health in the era of the SDGs while at the same time evacuating pleasure, a cornerstone and fundamental aspect of human sexuality, so completely?

Problematizing national sexual health strategies in Europe

The idea that sexual health has a plurality of usages and a broad field of impact is not a novel viewpoint. Most clearly formulated by Epstein and Mamo (2017), in their statement that

> because paring "sexual" with "health" serves to legitimize and sanitize sexuality, the framing of sexual issues as matters of sexual health is widely appealing across multiple social areas, and this appeal helps to explain both the proliferation of the term and the diversification of its uses.
>
> (p. 176)

While we agree with Epstein and Mamo that sex is sanitized and legitimized through its coupling with health, we also want to bring this into contact with a more theoretically informed reading by way of Carol Bacchi (Bacchi, 2000, 2015; Bacchi & Goodwin, 2016) and Michel Foucault (1990a, 2001). We seek to investigate what the problem that sexual health seeks to address is and, through this perhaps mundane phrasing, we arrive at some of the same typologies that Epstein and Mamo did, with, however, a few important differences which we will come back to later in this chapter.

The question that this chapter seeks to engage with is: *What is it that the concept of sexual health tries to answer? What problems does sexual health seek to address and in what manner? In short, what is the problematization of sexual health when we see it emerge in various national sexual health strategies?* If, as Epstein and Mamo have stated, the polysemy of sexual health leads to a proliferation of the term in such a fashion that it comes to address several social issues at once, then what are the *problems* that these social issues seem to generate? Are these problems "sexual" in nature, or are they related to the notion of "health"?

We take as our main methodological and theoretical inspiration the concept of "problematization" as developed by Michel Foucault (2001). However, we also want to make use of the concept of problematization as reformulated by Carol Bacchi and her "what's the problem represented to be?" (WPR) approach to the analysis of political policies (Bacchi, 2000, 2009, 2012, 2015; Bacchi & Goodwin, 2016). Foucault states that the study of various practices should start from a study of "problematization," that is, asking, "how and why certain things (behavior, phenomena, processes) became a problem" (Foucault, 2001, p. 171). In investigating various problems, Foucault states that there is a certain double movement to the study of problematization; that is, one tries in the same analytical frame to "see how the different solutions to a problem have been constructed; but also, how these solutions result from a specific form of problematization" (Foucault, 1984, p. 389). As such, a starting point for us here in this chapter might be to think about the discourse of sexual health not only as a "solution" but indeed as a form of an answer to a problem, to the various problems that emerge when we combine sexuality and health under one rubric. However, we should be careful to think that sexual health as a public health concept is a banal answer to the *problem of sexuality and health*; rather, linking the concept of problematization to the discourse of sexual health does not mean just looking at it as a reply to a question, that is, *what to do about sexuality and health*. Rather, by problematizing what happens when we combine sexuality with health, we can see that sexual health not only becomes the answer to a certain set of problems but becomes itself a problem.

Problematization as Foucault used it can be seen as a method wherein problematization is "an object of analysis. For example, the process by which modes of living or modes of self-care become problems is what is meant by problematization."[1] In this form, problematization is seen through the by now well-known formulation made by Foucault that problematization is the name given to the development of a genealogy of problems; "Why a problem and why such a kind of problem, why a certain way of problematizing appears at a given point in time" (Foucault et al., 2007, p. 141). In linking this to Foucault's terms, we can look at a quote where he states that, for him, one of the ways the concept of problematization works is by the work it does to

> rediscover at the root of these diverse solutions the general form of problematization that has been made them possible – even in their very opposition; or what has made possible the transformations of the difficulties and obstacles of a practice into a general problem for which one proposes diverse practical solutions. It is problematization that responds to these difficulties, but by doing something quite other than expressing them or manifesting them: in connection with them it develops the conditions in which possible response will be given; it defines the elements that will constitute what the different solutions attempt to respond to. This development of a given into a question, this transformation of a group of obstacles and difficulties into problems to which the diverse solutions will attempt to produce a response, this is what constitutes the point of problematization and the specific work of thought.
>
> (Rabinow, 1984, p. 389)

This is part of the project of this chapter: to look at how the discourse of sexual health in public health policies is seen as a solution to a problem, that is, sexuality and health, but at the same time *becomes* its problematization; that is, the very term "sexual health" invokes certain solutions to the problem of sexuality and health which in themselves are also elements that should not be seen as the final solution to an issue – rather they are contingent and themselves open to critical analysis for the productive work they do. Furthermore, this chapter also responds to the question of what kind of obstacles the discourse of sexual health aims at transforming, removing, or controlling concerning sexual health policies. How are the solutions proposed under such a regime, or rather, under such a problematization, also in and of themselves problematic?

In short, this chapter will seek to answer how the concept of sexual health as seen in the post-SDG era allows for a problematization of sexuality and health which goes beyond the issues of sexuality and health. In this chapter, we will focus on six national strategies and action plans across five European nations and how these open up governance of sexual health which goes beyond addressing sexuality and health. The six nations we have looked at in this chapter are Norway, Ireland, England, Sweden, Denmark, and France. What all of these strategies have in common is that they all were formed *after* the SDG Agenda in 2015 and that they also directly refer to and play on the SDG Agenda and the notion of sustainable development goals. The UN and WHO have highlighted the need for and use of harmonized sexual health strategies that address reproductive and sexual health issues within the same strategy (WHO, 2016). This is also another key commonality that these six nations and their sexual health plans have in common: they have all answered this call for harmonized sexual health plans.

How to analyze sexual health in policy and action plans: a few words on methods

We took as our departure point six national action plans or policy strategies that addressed sexuality. The national plans we looked at were Norway and its national strategy for sexual health called "Snakk om det!" [Talk about it!] (Ministry of Health and Social Services Norway, 2017); Public Health England (PHE) and its *Health Promotion for Sexual and Reproductive Health and HIV* (Public Health England, 2015); the Danish national sexual health plan, "Seksuel sundhed" [Sexual health] (Sunhedsstyrelsen, 2018); the French *National Sexual Health Strategy* from 2017 (Ministry of Solidarity and Health, France, 2017); the current Swedish "knowledge review" of sexual health services and the state of the art in Sweden, which is to serve as the foundation upon which a forthcoming national sexual health strategy will be built in 2020/2021; and, finally, the *National Sexual Health Strategy* for Ireland from 2015 (An Roinn Siainte, 2015). We also included the WHO European Region's *Action Plan for Sexual and Reproductive Health. Towards Achieving the 2030 Agenda for Sustainable Development in Europe – Leaving No One Behind* (WHO, 2016). We chose these seven documents based on the following rationale: (i) they all respond to or cite a focus on the SDGs as a framework for understanding and including sexual health as a broad way of understanding health linked to sexuality and reproduction; (ii) all of them follow and cite the need for a broad definition of sexual health per the WHO definition and the UN's usage of the term (WHO, 2002); and (iii) finally, they were all produced in the wake of, or close to, the UN's launch of the SDGs and subsequent rollout of the Agenda 2030 document in 2015 (UN, 2015).

We wanted to identify what sexual health meant in each of these national strategies and plans by asking "What are the problems that the concept of sexual health seeks to address?" and "how and why certain things (behavior, phenomena, processes) became a problem" (Foucault, 2001, p. 171). In investigating various problems, Foucault states that there is a certain double movement to the study of problematization; that is, one tries in the same analytical frame to "see how the different solutions to a problem have been constructed; but also, how these solutions result from a specific form of problematization" (1984, p. 389). As such, a starting point for us here in this chapter might be to think about the discourse of sexual health not as a "solution" but indeed as a form of an answer to a problem, but not just the answer to *one problem* but many, as we will argue. We will implicitly argue that the problem of sexuality in connection to health can be seen as the practical context for thinking about the problem of sex, of intimacy. It is about the ordering of knowledge about human intimacy, how to know it, to account for it, and to control it. It's about answering the perceived problem of sex and its relationship to human behavior, conduct, and practice. This becomes more problematic when, as we will see later on, the role of pleasure and well-being seems to be all but absent in all of the strategies we analyzed. In the SDG era, the knowledge that is being produced and focused on when it comes to sexual health is knowledge about pedagogy, biomedicine, and legal rights. While we do not argue that these aspects are trivial or not welcome, we argue that knowledge about pleasure as part of health, as part of human sexuality, is avoided to such a degree that it might be difficult to talk about sustainable sexual health if we avoid one of the fundamental aspects of human sexuality: pleasure.

If we agree that the focus on sexual health represents a proposed "solution" to not just one problem but many problems, including HIV/AIDS, STIs, reproduction, and issues of identity and rights, then the "problematization" of sexual health as it appears in these documents represents a dual object of analysis; on the one hand, sexual health is seen as the "solution" to the issue of, for instance, HIV/AIDS or sexual rights. However, on the other hand, sexual health and its implementation *become a problem*. This duality is produced, as Bacchi states, through a double movement wherein the issue under analysis becomes both an "answer" to a problem *and a problem in and of itself through problematization*. For Bacchi, the concept of problematization as it is used within her methodology offers a way of discerning how governmental practices, understood broadly, produce "problems" as particular kinds of problems, and, alongside and through the production of "problems," governmental practices contribute to the production of "subjects," "objects," and "places" (Bacchi & Goodwin, 2016, p. 14). As for Foucault, so for Bacchi; problematization can be seen as functioning dually: on the one hand, it can be seen as a form of critical analysis, that is, putting something into question, but, on the other hand, it can also signal a shift of focus onto the products of governmental practices, that is, how issues are problematized (Bacchi & Goodwin, 2016, p. 16). Nikolas Rose and Peter Miller, scholars whose work falls perhaps within the rubric of "governmentality studies," state that government or governmentality is a "problematizing activity" (2017, p. 181). In this sense, the use of policy within modern nation-states relies on, as Osborne states, a functioning of policy wherein "policy cannot get to work without first problematizing its territory" (1997, p. 174). In short, following Bacchi but also Foucault to a certain extent, to intervene in people's lives through policy, the state first needs to target something as a problem that needs fixing. This could be "poverty," "obesity," "suicide," or, in this case, "sexual health." This way of analyzing various policy problems within the art of government states that policies or other state interventions "*produce* 'problems' as particular sorts of problems. Further, it is argued that how these 'problems' are constituted shape lives and worlds" (Bacchi & Goodwin, 2016, p. 16). Analytically, this has value, for it opens up the fact that, for sexual health and the broad focus it has garnered in the post-SDG world, a sort of "answer" to the many "problems" associated with the combination of sexuality and health can be opened and critically examined not for its intentions to "ensure a sustainable future" but to allow us to see the *effects, processes, manners of conducting oneself and others in the name of "sexual health" and how the issues surrounding sexual health are framed.* Thus, analytical focus is moved from "result," that is, the "answer to the problem" onto how the problem came about, what effects its *answer* has produced, and how people respond not to the focus on sexual health per se but rather to the many processes that are being animated through this calling for an intensification of sexual health policies and action plans.

This also brings us to the issue of why we analyze policy texts in this chapter. Following Bacchi's reformulation of Foucault's work on various texts, we follow Bacchi's call when she states that to undertake "this kind of analysis Foucault recommends starting from 'practical texts,'" "the supposedly minor texts of those who made policy and wielded power" (Bacchi & Goodwin, 2016, p. 34). The reason is that "These policy texts, he tells us, introduce 'programmes of conduct'" (Bacchi & Goodwin, 2016, p. 34), which, per Foucault, are "written for the purpose of offering rules, opinion, and advice on how to behave as one should." As such, they are "objects of a 'practice'" intended to "constitute the eventual framework of everyday conduct" (Foucault, 2012, pp. 11–12). This is precisely the reason we have chosen to work within the framework of problematization in analyzing these sexual health policies; we see them as just these kinds of "prescriptive texts" mentioned by Bacchi and Foucault. In this fashion, this framework "questions the WPR [Carol Bacchi's analytical reorientation of Foucault] approach brings to 'practical texts' make it possible to identify and interrogate governmental problematizations via these understandings of practices, events, and relations" (Bacchi & Goodwin, 2016, p. 34). Understanding policy texts in this fashion offer us a way of looking at them as texts that function as just that, a prescriptive set of texts that relies on a particular problematization (Bacchi, 2012, p. 4). Following this logic, Bacchi states that we can "work backward" to deduce how it produces a "problem" (Bacchi, 2012, p. 4). Our link to this kind of analysis of policy documents lies in looking at the policy text analyzed here as sites wherein sexual health plans become the solution to a set of different problems (HIV/AIDS, infertility, sexual rights, and even sustainable development) but also become *themselves a problem*: how to "end AIDS," how to "ensure sexual rights," "how to minimize irresponsible sexual behavior," and so on.

Preventing sexually transmitted infections and HIV in the name of health and sustainability

The first and perhaps most central social aspect of the concept of sexual health as it emerges in the policy plans we have analyzed relates to the prevention of STIs, including HIV/AIDS. In this framing of sexual health, a focus on sexual health implies the solution to the spread of STIs such as HIV through "programs of surveillance, prevention, or treatment of sexually transmitted infections" (Epstein & Mamo, 2017, p. 181). Following the "what's the problem represented to be?" analysis of Bacchi, we could state that this framing of sexual health sees sexual health policies as the solution to the "problem" of disease spreading and its associated mortality and morbidity rates. It also creates two forms of obligations: one which obligates state organizations (and others) and another which obligates individuals. Combining the insights from Epstein and Mamo with that of the problematization framework of Bacchi and Foucault, the policy plans frame institutional obligations as pertaining to the creation of preventive campaigns and the implementation of monitoring and epidemiological surveillance technologies such as the use of indicators; the collection of epidemiological data through STI tests; and the obligation to, at each level of governance, create STI preventive services.

A case in point here could be the following excerpt from the Norwegian strategy plan, *Talk About It!* (Ministry of Health and Social Services Norway, 2017). Here the main goal of relating to STIs is framed as "a reduction in the prevalence of all sexually transmittable diseases" (Ministry of Health and Social Services Norway, 2017, p. 38). The plan then goes on to list the distribution of gonorrhea based on age, where the youngest man was 14 and the oldest was 77 years old. For women, the oldest individual with a gonorrhea infection was 69 (Ministry of Health and Social Services Norway, 2017, p. 38). It then states that while most new infections occur amongst young men who have sex with other men, the data shows that even older adults, both female and male, regardless of sexual orientation, are at risk of gonorrhea (Ministry of Health and Social Services Norway, 2017, p. 38). The text concludes that based on this, that is, gonorrhea as a proxy for STI prevalence amongst *all* ages and *all* groups, there is an evident need for visible information campaigns and dissemination of knowledge of prevention and that this information should be aimed at "all age groups and genders, and that testing services for STIs are easily accessible to all" (Ministry of Health and Social Services Norway, 2017, p. 38). To reach the goal of a reduction of all STIs and their prevalence within the Norwegian population, the document suggests, amongst other things, an "increase in measurements to increase condom usage in all population groups," as well as "the development of positive attitudes to condom usage, easy access to condoms, and training in proper condom usage" (Ministry of Health and Social Services Norway, 2017, p. 39). Furthermore, sexual education and sexual health campaigns aimed at focusing on positive experiences with condom usage and training in sexual communication and negotiation skills that secure safe sex are important (Ministry of Health and Social Services Norway, 2017, p. 39).

In the previous, we can see that sexual health within this framing focuses on sexuality as being a "practice of potential risk" (Epstein & Mamo, 2017, p. 181), while health is framed as reducing risk through strategies such as condom usage, the uptake of knowledge about safe sex, and the use of this knowledge. The individual injunction is to engage in responsible sexual practices which are predicated upon the proper use of condoms and the use of communication and knowledge skills that are meant to minimize risk. On the institutional level, the policy plan sets up an obligation for various health care authorities to (i) secure good access to condoms in general and in particular within areas with a high risk of infections, (ii) roll out condom campaigns aimed at population groups at particularly high risk of STI infections, (iii) secure a high level of human papillomavirus (HPV) vaccination coverage through national vaccination programs while also offering vaccines to groups with an elevated risk of infection, (iv) secure access to testing at a diverse range of testing sites and offer in co-operation with NGOs, (v) consider pilot projects for at-home testing for STIs and the possibility for digital correspondence and consultations when tests are positive, and, finally, (vi) implement PrEP to reduce the number of new HIV infections (Ministry of Health and Social Services Norway, 2017, p. 42). These responses to the *problem of STIs* can be retrofitted by arguments made earlier in the report. Before listing these "solutions" to the problem of STIs, the document lists, amongst the keys to lowering STI infections, HIV included, those that involve "increased testing activity," "anonymous testing," "early detection and treatment of STIs, including HIV," and "information campaigns aimed at groups at elevated risk" (Ministry of Health and Social Services Norway, 2017, pp. 40–41).

Now, responding to the theoretical framework we have used, the previous excerpts show that sexual health in this frame is predicated upon risk reduction and an obligation by institutions to secure and implement a range of surveillance techniques, which is further highlighted by page 55, on which the report states the importance of and need for "better and more granular forms of data" which " can monitor both STIs" and "the knowledge on sexual health and STIs" through various forms of data surveillance, e-health campaigns included (Ministry of Health and Social Services Norway, 2017, p. 55). These obligations are thus laid at the feet of various governmental actors and levels ranging from municipalities to state-run agencies.

At the same time, sexual health as it is connected to STIs obligates individuals. While the report states, as we have seen, that "everybody" is a potential risk, as envisioned by the large age spread in the proxy STI of gonorrhea, the strategy does create subjects and even spaces wherein risk is distributed differently, and thus so is responsibility. Men who have sex with men are mentioned as one such differential risk group; the same pertains to immigrants. Services and measures to reach people who "for various reasons don't get tested" (Ministry of Health and Social Services Norway, 2017, p. 41) are mentioned as being of "particular importance" (Ministry of Health and Social Services Norway, 2017, p. 41). Furthermore, men who have sex with men have, the report states, higher use of legal and illegal drugs in combination with casual and unprotected sex, which in turn gives a higher risk of infection of all types of sexually transmitted diseases (Ministry of Health and Social Services Norway, 2017, p. 40). The problematization of sexual health in this frame not only allows for addressing and talking about sexuality and health but indeed drug use and its link to STIs. The subject positions that are being enacted in this frame are a subject wherein, while potentially being all of "us," in fact, more and more, "the burdens and benefits of epidemiological surveillance are not evenly distributed but instead fall heavily on particular groups" (Epstein, 1995, p. 182), in this case, young men who have sex with men, immigrants, and, to a certain degree, young adults, as is the case with Chlamydia, where both men and women in the age bracket 15 to 24 years are highlighted as being at particular risk (Ministry of Health and Social Services Norway, 2017, p. 37). Certain subjects are created which are "at elevated risk" and thus also disproportionally targeted by behavior campaigns aimed at teaching the subject "bodily scrutiny" and "risk calculations" with regard to their sexual health, a body that is "permeable and vulnerable; an at-risk self that is also potentially amendable to education and self-regulation" (Epstein & Mamo, 2017, p. 182), which is also at the same time the target of various biomedical interventions and surveillance techniques such as PrEP, STI testing, and, if positive, treatment. It also creates spaces of risk as envisioned by the statement of "secure good access to condoms in general and in particular within areas with a high risk of infections," a clear differentiation of risk based on geographical location.

This kind of logic is also traceable in all of the other sexual health strategies. A case in point would be the French *National Sexual Health Strategy* (Ministry of Solidarity and Health, France, 2017). In the French case, the strategy is divided into six priority areas, which in turn are subdivided into a total of twenty aims, which are further divided into visions, priorities, and targets to be reached by 2023. Priority II directly addresses the question of sexual health as framed through a focus on STIs, prevention, screening, and treatment (Ministry of Solidarity and Health, France, 2017, p. 20). Amongst the targets for this priority is "in 2020, 95% of people living with HIV are aware of their HIV status"; "in 2020, 95% of all people tested who are infected with HIV receive the recommended antiretroviral treatment"; "in 2020, 95% of people receiving anti-retroviral treatment have a lasting undetectable viral load"; "in 2023, 75% of adolescents covered by the hepatitis B vaccination (95% in 2030); in 2023, 60% of adolescents covered by the HPV vaccination (80% in 2030); reduce the incidence of the most common and serious STIs" (Ministry of Solidarity and Health France, 2017, p. 20). These targets for the French plan are aligned with the *programmatic time* of the UNAIDS goals of "ending AIDS" in 2020 (UNAIDS, 2017, 2014) by focusing on the so-called "90–90–90" targets. The 90–90–90 targets stipulate that "90% of people living with

HIV know their HIV status; 90% of people who know their status receive treat-ment; 90% of people on HIV treatment have a suppressed viral load" (UNAIDS, 2014). The 90–90–90 targets have since then become part of many nations' public health response to ending AIDS. Many nations now use these indicators as a way of reporting progress on ending AIDS and thus also fulfilling the global "promise" made in the UN SDGs on "ending AIDS" and ensuring an "HIV free generation" (UNAIDS, 2019). UNAIDS states that, "When this three-part target is achieved, at least 73% of all people living with HIV worldwide will be virally suppressed – a two- to three-fold increase over current rough estimates of viral suppression" (UNAIDS, 2014, p. 3). It also aligns itself with the programmatic time of the UN's SDG targets by referencing the 2030 Agenda timeline (UN, 2015). However, by focusing on these targets, the strategy also frames sexual health in this niche as an injunction to various governmental agencies to roll out "test, treat, and retain pro-grams, while also creating on obligation on the individual level to get tested, and if testing positive, access and adhere to antiretroviral treatment to reach 'unde-tectable'." There's also the issue of which subjects are created here; by framing sexual health in this fashion, the risk is highlighted as well as bodily scrutiny and engagement with testing and treatment regimes. It also creates normative and quantifiable metrics for "success" in terms of HIV as part of sexual health; sub-jects are to, at any given time, know their status, to become "undetectable," and to adhere to treatment. For HPV, the obligation is to get vaccinated. While uptake and access to ARVs for HIV and vaccines against HPV are important in both reducing new cases and reducing mortality and morbidity rates from HIV and cancers, the point of this is to highlight how sexual health is also highly predicated upon what has been called the pharmaceuticalization and biomedicalization of sexual health (Abraham, 2010; Bell & Figert, 2012; Biehl, 2007; Meneu, 2018). Sexual health and the reduction of STIs in this refraction of the problem become highly contingent upon biomedical pharmaceuticals as a solution.

However, as Bacchi and Goodwin state, one way of problematizing any policy document is to ask what is being left silent and how we can conceptualize the issue differently, or, rather, what is left unspoken (2016, p. 22)? A case in point here would be: Why these numerical figures? What about those who do not know their status, maintain and access treatment, or reach undetectable viral load lev-els? These "silent" discursive subjects are not mentioned in the document, and thus the document also produces a set of subjectivities that are only mentioned in the negative; that is, they are only defined in their absence. Yet they are still subjects that are being produced as "lacking" or "not counted." Silence within the realm of policy documents about sexual health should not then be seen as "less the absolute limit of discourse, the other side from which it is separated by a strict boundary, than an element that functions alongside the things said, with them and in relation to them within over-all strategies" (Foucault, 1990a, p. 27). The delineated subjects produced by the number "95%," "75%," or "60%" produce clear goals to be reached but also clearly demarcate populations to be targeted by various state actions in the name of sexual health. Yet the populations that remain "left behind," that is, the "5%" or the "25%," do not exist outside of discourse;

rather, they are integral to the production and the possibility of conceptualizing those targeted by, as we have seen, a host of screening, testing, preventing, and treating initiatives.

The policy document follows along much the same lines as the Norwegian one in terms of focusing on new ways of screening and testing for STIs. Aim 3 within Priority II states, for instance, that one of the key goals of better screening of "key populations" is to "develop methods to encourage population groups who are the latest to come for screening to do so (men born in sub-Saharan Africa for HIV and HBV in particular) and who are most unaware of their status" (Ministry of Solidarity and Health France, 2017, p. 24). Another key screening injunction which is addressed to both various health providers and individuals is to "encourage the use of self-test for HIV screening" (Ministry of Solidarity and Health France, 2017, p. 24). This was, as we have seen, addressed in the Norwegian context, where it was to be evaluated as a screening tool for reaching "at-risk populations." It is also mentioned in the strategic plan developed by Public Health England (PHE, 2015, p. 18). By highlighting the need for and scale-up of self-testing for HIV, these sexual health policies set in motion screening outside of the clinic, as several scholars have pointed to (Banda, 2015; Lupton, 2012, 2013a, 2013b, 2015). While self-test kits for the diagnosis of HIV have been seen as a welcome new addition to HIV screening as well as being part of a more personalized focus on HIV testing and prevention (Choko et al., 2011; Jantarapakde et al., 2018), they have also been linked to the rise of an "individualization" of risk and responsibility, as Banda argued (2015). Furthermore, the issue of "at-home testing kits" for HIV has also been problematized as a potential coercive technology wherein people are forced by others to test for HIV (Banda, 2015; Walensky & Paltiel, 2006). While seen by some as a liberating and useful technology of screening which also allows the user to test in the "comfort of their own home," as OraQuick, one of the largest producers of at-home testing kits, states on its webpage,[2] it has also been seen as threat which might undermine HIV efforts if the price point of the self-testing kit is too high, and it plays on neo-liberal ideas of responsibility, risk calculations, and market choice logics, which makes responsibility individualized, since health prevention is now more and more located outside the clinic (Kenworthy et al., 2018; Sandset, 2019). Returning to the French strategy, there's also a case to be made for sexual health as catering to the production of "at risk" subjects in Priority IV, "Meet the specific needs of the most vulnerable populations" (Ministry of Solidarity and Health France, 2017, p. 33). Sexual health here is once again linked to and allows for a discourse that plays on risk and risk reduction through testing, self-scrutiny, and state interventions such as testing, treating, and vaccination programs. However, here the strategy also distributes risk by creating populations that are at "excessive risk," that is, "groups with widespread prevalence" such as LGBTI individuals (Ministry of Solidarity and Health France, 2017, p. 34). However, it also produces people who are at elevated risk due to their *perceived lack of risk*, that is, seniors and people with disabilities (Ministry of Solidarity and Health France, 2017, p. 34). While the Norwegian strategy produced risk across all population groups and genders by recourse to proxy numbers of the youngest to oldest incidents of gonorrhea, the French strategy interpellates both *high-risk individuals by widespread prevalence while at the same time also producing risk in seniors and people with disabilities due to* "under-estimates of exposure to risks" (Ministry of Solidarity and Health France, 2017, p. 34). In an interesting mechanism, underestimates of sexual health risks lead to risk: the groups in question become targets of risk interventions not due to their alleged high-risk prevalence but because the numbers point to underestimates. In a way, silence here is productive in the Foucauldian sense in that underestimates, that is, blind spots in the epidemiological data, produce people at risk, since the silence of the data points to the presence of risk that one perceives as being there yet has not yet clearly identified. This production of "at-risk subjects" through too little data or underestimates has also been observed in relation to same-sex–attracted women and sexual health as framed by the risk of STIs. Here, the case is that same-sex–attracted women are at risk precisely since they do not show up in studies on STI risks. A direct case from our material would be the Norwegian strategy which states that

> expectations to certain groups' sexual behaviors might result in misunderstandings in terms of health care advice. For example, same-sex attracted women have received information from health care personnel that they are not amongst the target population for the screening program for cervical cancer due to their sexual orientation.
> (Ministry of Health and Social Services Norway, 2017, p. 28)

Risk is here constructed through the risk that *blind spots* bring, that is, that underestimates in risk are due to misunderstandings, a lack of knowledge, and omissions in the epidemiological network. In this way, the risk becomes something akin to the now perhaps notorious statement made by then-Secretary of State Donald Rumsfeld, who (in)famously was quoted saying, "as we know, there are known knowns; there are things we know we know. We also know there are known unknowns; that is to say, we know there are some things we do not know. But there are also unknown unknowns – the ones we don't know we don't know."[3] While Rumsfeld's statement was made in relation to the "war on terror" and the subsequent policy of "preemption," the fact that these reports also create subjects who are at risk due to their perceived *non-risk* can be seen as an epidemiological exercise in precisely uncovering the "unknown unknowns" of sexual health risks.

Going back to the French strategy, the connection between drug use and STI risk also becomes possible by talking about sexual health. The "incitement to discourse" of Foucault (Epstein, 2003; Foucault, 1990a) allows for, as we have argued earlier, an extended field of impact wherein sexual health policies allow the inclusion of a multitude of meanings associated with sexuality and health to emerge. As in the Norwegian context, the French strategy also includes a focus on drug use, sex, and health when it states that one of the most pressing issues in intensifying prevention, screening, and access to rights and care for populations that are most exposed to HIV, HPV, hepatitis C virus (HCV), and STIs is to "develop an overall sexual health strategy that takes into account mental health, other chronic diseases, and the reduction of risks and damages related to addiction" (Ministry of Solidarity and Health France, 2017, p. 36). Furthermore, this involves working to reduce the risks and damages related to practices that involve consuming psychoactive substances in a sexual context ("chemsex") in that they "maintain the dynamic of the HIV epidemic and to the increase of HCV infections in the homosexual population" (Ministry of Solidarity and Health France, 2017, p. 34). This is also found in Public Health England's strategy wherein MSM are targeted by the same connection between HIV/HCV, drug use (chemsex), and sexuality and health when the strategy states that one of its main objectives is "to reduce the proportion reporting use of harmful illicit substances, including a reduction in the proportion reporting 'chemsex' or steroid abuse" (Public Health England, 2015, p. 17). In both cases, sexual health becomes a way of talking about and targeting drug use as one important risk factor. However, it also explicitly produces a particular group that needs risk reduction interventions: MSM or "a homosexual population," as the French wording goes. Following Bacchi and her problematization, this kind of production of specific subject positions within the policy document creates subjects that can be targeted by specific interventions, while at the same time, these very same subjects also become obligated to conduct themselves according to various sexual health regimes in order to reduce their own risk but also the "dynamic of the HIV epidemic," for instance. Sexual health in this frame allows for the enactment of subjects that are in need of interventions that target not only intimacies and health but addiction issues and thus either harm reduction strategies or prohibiting/reducing total usage of, for instance, chemsex drugs. There is a case to be made in this for a subtle nuance within the French and English documents wherein the French document seems to be calling for harm reduction, while the English document seems to be calling for a flat-out reduction of the phenomena of chemsex. This subtle nuance is important inasmuch as there is a qualitative difference between trying to reduce a drug practice through a focus on the total number of people reporting usage and, on the other hand, working to reduce the effects of usage, that is, a harm reduction strategy that aims at not reducing the total number of reported users but rather the total number of unhealthy effects of said practice.

Once again, the silences that this sort of rhetoric also produces are interesting; while the rise of chemsex as a social and medical phenomenon related to gay male sexuality has had an almost perennial explosion, as envisioned by both research literature and exposure in the popular press,[4] how chemsex becomes first and foremost a "gay" problem is seen in these policy documents. The silences of heterosexual use of drugs in combination with sex are all but omitted in these documents, thus framing drug use in relation to sexual health as an issue within gay communities which is thus in need of health intervention in the name of sustainable sexual health. Heterosexual chemsex is, as stated, not mentioned in any of the policy papers analyzed, even though the use of psychoactive drugs within heterosexual or straight settings exists, as envisioned by a recent BMJ blogpost with subsequent references to chemsex amongst heterosexual people.[5]

Without going too far, the focus on chemsex as a "gay" problem is not new, as attested to by Steven Epstein's work covering the earlier days of the AIDS epidemic. Here the blame for the epidemic was often referred to by way of focusing on gay men's usage of "poppers" and their combination with a party culture perceived as promiscuous (Epstein, 1996). Newer research has pointed out that the framing of chemsex as a "gay" problem omits the fact that heterosexuals also engage in the use of psychoactive drugs and sex and that the role of alcohol in relation to sexual health is often omitted entirely. Some researchers have dubbed the emerging focus on chemsex as a "re-crising" of gay male sexuality through a moral panic that focuses on promiscuous sex, irresponsible sexual behavior, and total neglect of one's health and even productivity (Hakim, 2017; Lovelock, 2018). As a final component to this, the only policy paper in our pool that directly addressed alcohol and the role of sexual health risk was the Irish National Sexual Health plan, but even here, alcohol is spuriously connected to an increase in sexual health risk, and the relationship between alcohol and sexual risk-taking is deemed "not clear cut" (An Roinn Siainte, 2015, p. 36). As such, in this enactment of sexuality and health, sexual health allows one to address drug use and addiction, allowing for a much broader field of impact and thus also for targeted populations to be interpellated. Sexual health, it seems, can be concerned with a plethora of social issues, amongst these drug use. However, drug use only marks gay male sexuality as its object of problematization in these policy documents, thus absolving heterosexual populations of the issue of linking sexual health to drug use. What implications this has for health services should be investigated in full, but it does seem that the policy papers thus far analyzed set up services and interventions that are mainly targeting gay men in relation to the issue of sexual health risk and drug use.

Sexual function, pharma, and subjectivities

While screening, preventing, and treating STIs and HIV have become well-known staples in sexual health policy papers, the inclusion of sexual dysfunction and sexual function, in general, seems to have been a more recent development, which, as Giami, alongside Epstein and Mamo, states, has coincided with the development of "sexual medicine," which emerged in the 1970s (Epstein & Mamo, 2017; Giami, 2002). However, the inclusion of sexual function as part of public health policies such as the ones we have analyzed here should also be seen in relation to how we have charted out the developments within the very concept of sexual health. Finally, the inclusion of sexual dysfunction as a problem for public health should be seen as a result of the entanglements between biopharmaceuticals such as the launch of Viagra in 1998 (Epstein & Mamo, 2017, p. 183), the focus on holistic sexual health, and the emergence of a focus on person-centered care. If we continue to follow the methodological reading of our material as we have done so far, a way of framing the issue of the inclusion of sexual dysfunction within these policy papers is to ask: "What are the problems that sexual dysfunction is said to represent?", "What sorts of subject positions are produced through the connection between sexuality and dysfunction?", and "What sort of other aspects of health, if any, are talked about through a focus on dysfunction?"

We can start by looking at a few excerpts from the material at hand. First of all, sexual dysfunction in sexual health strategies can be divided into three main lines of problems; the first one concerns female infertility. The second lies within male erectile dysfunction and subsequent intimacy issues. Finally, the third is conceptualized as pertaining to "pain and discomfort" during intercourse for both men and women. An example of the first, that is, female infertility, can be drawn from the WHO European Regional Office Action Plan, wherein we can read that Objective 2.5 in this strategy is to "inform people about the adverse effect of advancing age on fertility" and "promot[e] actions to prevent infertility, such as prevention of obesity and unsafe abortions" (WHO, 2016, p. 12). A similar theme can be discerned in the Danish document, where we read that the number of women who are registered at a Danish address and with a male partner who are receiving fertility treatment has been stable at around 10,000 to 11,000 women a year. Furthermore, the main reason for infertility amongst women but also men is increased age, here defined as 35 years for women and 40 years for men. Finally, the section also states that STIs and a broad range of lifestyle diseases also contribute to infertility amongst both men and women, such as smoking and obesity (Sunhedsstyrelsen, 2018, p. 7). A final example on this kind of problematization of fertility when linked to sexual health comes from the French strategy, which states that one of its many aims is to

> include infertility prevention among men and women in relation to behavioral detriments (being overweight/underweight, tobacco and alcohol consumption) in national plans . . . preserve the natural fertility of women and men by strengthening and adapting methods of communication (information on periods of fertility, contraception options, birth spacing, consequences of undiagnosed STIs).
>
> (Ministry of Solidarity and Health France, 2017, p. 32)

Fertility in these extracts can be analyzed according to the ways in which they produce "answers to problems" as well as how they frame these problems. We also can see these documents as creating, as we have stated, various subject positions from where the policy documents can and do create subjects that can be governed and governed in a specific way. Finally, the documents also show how fertility, when it emerges within the field of sexual health writ large, allows for policymakers to address other issues besides just sexual health; in this case, the action plans not only address sexual health but indeed obesity, underweight, and smoking as ways of problematizing fertility. By invoking these other social issues, the implicit understanding is that infertility will also be reduced; thus, the answer to the problem of infertility is located outside the realm of sexuality proper. Perhaps it is better to state that the realm of sexual health, in this case, is extended into other health realms such as nutrition, weight management, and smoking cessation? Regardless, the point that we have made seems to hold true; sexual health, through how it is framed and developed in the era of the SDGs, allows for interventions beyond the field of sexuality and is linked to a much greater degree to a holistic framework, encompassing a diverse field of problems.

Sexual health in the age of sustainability is, as we have seen, a more holistic rendition of the term that it was in the earlier years. The upside of this is that the very term allows us to see health and well-being as holistic, yet the potential downside is that sexual health becomes a pivot point for intervening in other health issues as well as rendering human sexuality as being always also predicated upon such a broad range of concepts that the drive for health optimization becomes all encompassing.

With regard to female infertility, it is also worth noting the framing in the Danish strategy which highlights the fact that statistics on women in fertility treatment services are linked to having a Danish address but, more so, also to living with a male partner. Following the idea of how these policy papers operate with silences and how these silences are productive, we can state that such a framing, first of all, relies on a heteronormative construction of the reproductive coupling between a woman and a man. The silence that is produced is how reproductive services thus seem to erase or at least mute the connection between same-sex–attracted women who want to enter into fertility treatments.

Another issue with how the framing of female infertility can be seen as problematic is how all of the reports to a large degree highlight not only the adoption of "healthy lifestyles" but also old age as the most important cause of female infertility. Choice is here invoked, and women waiting longer to have children is conjured up as a matter of lack of information on the difficulties that "birth spacing," or waiting "too long," will create problems with fertility. While our analysis is not contesting the fact that delaying reproduction is an issue, what is more problematic is the omission of *why* women in Europe wait longer to have children.

To wait "too long" is within the frames of the sexual health plans that we have analyzed, never put into the broader context of *why* women *choose* to have children later now than before. In the biopolitics of birth rates and reproduction, sexual health becomes a matter of state concern as falling birth rates become a concern of productivity and thus also the "health of the body politic." However, in these policies, there is no discussion of the structural and social incentives of having children at the *right time*, nor is there any debate about the structural barriers to having children. As Shammas and Sandset have noted in a similar setting:

> There is little or no discussion on interventions in the housing and labor market, even though some of the fundamental constraints on fertility rates spring from what Giddens termed "ontological insecurity", which has only risen with flexibilised labor relations and upwardly spiraling housing costs.
> (Giddens, 2013; Shammas & Sandset, 2020, p. 9)

As such, in these policy documents, fertility as part of sexual health is reduced and atomized to only focus on the individual (female) body, thus foreclosing any discussion of the structural barriers and fundamentally social aspects of human fertility. This "precludes any consolidated decommodifying interventions into the economic life of ordinary citizens. The structural and political instruments capable of redressing demographic problems are excluded at the level of ideology" (Shammas & Sandset, 2020, p. 9). Responsibility is thus leveled at the individual woman, who is interpellated into a subject position of a rational actor who, if only given enough information about "reproductive timing" will be able to procreate at a sort of optimal moment in the individual's life. Broader ideological issues are left outside of this refraction of sexual and reproductive health. There is no social "outside" to this discourse, and how infertility due to age is framed seems to be a "problem of choice" and not of social determinants or factors such as women's participation in higher education, career and work issues, structural factors such as various national mechanisms for child support, day-care pricing, and general welfare benefits that may or may not be attainable for women across Europe.

Population control and the role of reproductive autonomy

As noted by Epstein and Mamo, although the contemporary discourse of sexual health presumes the historical disentangling of the procreative and erotic aspects of people's lives, sexual and reproductive concerns have been linked ever since the time of the WHO definition (2017, p. 182). The current climate of the SDGs has even spurred an explicit discourse of *entanglement* of the sexual and the reproductive. We have argued earlier that this entanglement between the reproductive and the sexual in fact can be genealogically traced back to Malthus, and as such, it is little wonder that one of the key components of the sexual health strategies that we have looked at includes a section of what we have called "population control and the role of reproductive autonomy."

We can start by looking at the Norwegian strategy plan in order to look at how the issue of population control and reproductive autonomy is enacted in these strategies and reports. As with almost all of the reports we have analyzed, the refraction of reproductive health and autonomy is done through a focus on "reducing unwanted pregnancies and abortions." In the Norwegian report, the target goal of the government is "to prevent unwanted pregnancies among women of all ages" (Ministry of Health and Social Services Norway, 2017, p. 32). The report states that the main reason for a reduction of unwanted pregnancies is easy access to birth control technologies such as "the pill," spirals, and long-acting hormonal injections, as well as implants (Ministry of Health and Social Services Norway, 2017, p. 32).

Furthermore, the report adds that one of the most important initiatives in combination with access to birth control technologies is easy and accessible access to information and counseling on reproduction (Ministry of Health and Social Services Norway, 2017, pp. 11, 33). This is in particular highlighted in relation to the reduction of teen pregnancies and abortions. The report highlights that a key pillar in the reduction of unwanted pregnancies is to have school nurses available in each school so that both information about pregnancy as well as advice and information about access to birth control can be given to teenagers who are in school. One of the actions that the report suggests is to "enhance school nurses and midwifes and their roles in regards to the provision of birth control information as well as the administration of birth control to women" (Ministry of Health and Social Services Norway, 2017, p. 35). Much of the same sort of framing can be seen in the other strategies and reports. In the Swedish context, for instance, we can note that a rights perspective is much more prevalent than in the Norwegian strategy. In the Swedish report, it is noted that

> more concretely, good reproductive health involves, according to the UN, a responsible, satisfactory and safe sex life, the ability to reproduce, the freedom to decide when one wants to have children and one's ability to have healthy children. Good reproductive health is conditioned upon having the right knowledge and access to birth control technologies and protection against STIs in combination of having ensured access to safe condition under which to give birth.

The report goes on to note that to avoid unwanted pregnancies, it is paramount that women be given easy access to both birth control and information regarding pregnancies. There is an interesting difference between the Norwegian strategy and the Swedish in that the Swedish report states that "it is not a goal in and of itself to reduce abortions, rather the goal is to reduce unwanted pregnancies." Thus, the onus is not on abortions per se but rather to avoid unwanted pregnancies. Furthermore, it is of note that the Swedish report highlights three groups which it calls "priority target groups": "teenagers and young adults," "men and boys," and "vulnerable groups." This is different from the Norwegian context wherein men and boys, for instance, are omitted within the sections regarding pregnancies and abortions. While the Norwegian strategy seems to problematize unwanted pregnancies as a problem to be solved through biomedical technologies of prevention, information from health care workers, and the women themselves, the Swedish report includes men and boys as part of the problematization of unwanted pregnancies. That is, the report states that "these groups [men and boys] need to have more knowledge about and become more involved in discussions about how one avoids making someone pregnant who does not want to become pregnant or involuntarily become a parent." Men and boys in this context become part of the solution to the problem of unwanted pregnancies, which, in a sense, distributes responsibility beyond the usual focus on women and, to a certain degree, state provisions of ensuring that unwanted pregnancies are avoided.

Before making some analytical claims regarding this social niche as a way for the government to intervene in the intimate lives of its population in the name of "sustainable sexual health," let us look at the French and Irish strategies. Just like the other strategies we looked at, the French also included a section on what they named "Priority III – Improve reproductive health" (Ministry of Solidarity and Health France, 2017, p. 28). In this section, we can read the visions, priorities, and target indicators for 2023. One of the targets is to reduce the number of unwanted/unplanned pregnancies in women by one-third (Ministry of Solidarity and Health France, 2017, p. 28). Now, to do so, the report highlights that access to oral contraceptives is key, as is information regarding access to contraceptives and information regarding fertility and pregnancies. Furthermore, the strategy notes that female contraceptives are the dominant mode of birth control alongside condoms, yet male contraceptives are virtually absent from the market. Furthermore, the main reason for unwanted pregnancies was the failure of contraceptive technologies, such as condoms that break or women forgetting to adhere to the birth control pill (Ministry of Solidarity and Health France, 2017, p. 29). Finally, the strategy also highlights that there are large socioeconomic discrepancies in the use of contraception and that this is due to a lack of information and misrepresentation (Ministry of Solidarity and Health France, 2017, p. 29). In mentioning these aspects of reproductive health and autonomy, the strategy highlights the "biomedicalization" and even responsibilization of the female body through the consumption of oral contraceptives. Reproduction and autonomy seem to rest mainly within the realm of responsibility laid at the feet of women, except in the Swedish case, where men and boys, too, are interpellated as being part of this responsibilization of reproduction. The notion that it is often the female body that is being biomedicalized through contraception is a topic of much academic interest and analysis (Clarke et al., 2010; Mamo, 2003), as well as activist calls for a more even distribution of the contraceptive market and subsequent responsibility to develop male contraception on a par with female. In the previous, the French strategy highlights this explicitly, yet, as with all the other strategies, there are no calls for development or research into male contraception. Furthermore, sustainable sexual health, as it is refracted through the optic of reproductive control and autonomy, is primarily targeted at the female body and, in turn, the link between female bodies, biomedical solutions of reproductive control, and state information campaigns. Reproductive autonomy and control in this frame of analysis seem to locate responsibility across two actors: the women and the state. They also seem to equate autonomy with the market logic of choice of birth control inasmuch as the various strategies highlight choice as being linked to either condom usage, "the pill," hormonal coils, long-acting hormonal injections, and, finally, tubal ligation. These are, of course, bound to factors such as cost, knowledge about each technology of contraception, and access, a fact that is only mentioned as a barrier in terms of socioeconomic background. Now the French and Swedish highlight the discrepancies in access to and use of contraception and the link between socioeconomic status as well as age.

Sexual health as human rights: linking sexual health to rights and identity

Sexual health does not only focus on various biomedical aspects such as reproduction and sexual function, nor does it only focus on preventing STIs and HIV. Sexual health, as Epstein and Mamo note, has become a key term in which various rights aspects have been linked (2017). This can be seen in the SDG-era national sexual health strategies that we have analyzed. Sexual health is linked in many ways to various rights aspects such as the right to decide when to have children (reproductive autonomy), the right to decide when to have sex and corporal autonomy, and rights concerning LGBTQI communities. As such, sexual health has also become the a way of solving injustices linked to the *absence of sexual rights* (Epstein & Mamo, 2017, p. 180). In this refraction of the term "sexual health," health can be seen as a way of encouraging and supporting freedom from unwarranted external constraints or coercion, while the opposite would be subjugation and coercion and lack of rights, both in terms of reproductive rights and corporal autonomy but also the right to love without fear of social stigma or retribution.

In this analytical optic, sexual health has become linked to the term "sexual rights," a concept that in and of itself is emerging in the global health lexicon. Yet it is not without contestation. In the Norwegian strategy, it is stated that

> Good sexual health is predicated upon the individual's fulfillment of their sexual rights. Sexual rights are used in relation to human rights that ensure sexual and reproductive health. Central to these rights is the freedom to choose one's partner in accordance with one's sexual orientation, without being the victim of discrimination or criminalization. Other rights are those that pertain to the right to have sexual health education, right to and respect of bodily autonomy, freedom from violence, the right to choose when to have children and the right to choose to be sexually active. The concept of sexual rights are contested internationally but has broad social support in the Scandinavian countries and large parts of Europe.
>
> (Ministry of Health and Social Services Norway, 2017, p. 8).

In the previous, we see that sexual health is conceptually entangled with and predicated upon sexual rights. Sexual health is thus also always human rights in the optic. In the Norwegian, Swedish, and Danish strategies, this is clearly highlighted. In the Norwegian and Swedish strategies, large segments are dedicated to sexual rights as part of school curricula. Here the argument is that children and adolescents need to learn how to express themselves concerning sexuality and corporal autonomy. Learning to set boundaries is highlighted as key in teaching children and teenagers to respect other people's bodily autonomy, learning about boundary setting, and sexuality. Sexual health becomes predicated upon sexual rights, which in turn need to be learned and implemented from an early age in order to secure the individual.

This is also found in other plans in our analysis. In the WHO Strategy Plan for sexual and reproductive health, one of the founding visions of the strategy is to take actions such as "protecting, by legislative and other measures, people's rights related to sexual and reproductive health by eliminating discrimination and stigmatization" (2016, p. 7). In this view, sexual health is as much about rights and freedom from discrimination and stigma as it is about the biomedical aspects of sexual and reproductive health. Sexual rights are in themselves a rather broad category which includes gender equality rights, rights to equitable sexual health services, freedom from discrimination and stigma, and the right that protects individuals from gender and sexualized violence. In the WHO strategy for sexual and reproductive health, this is mentioned in the following actions to be taken by its member states: "awareness-raising, reinforcing the role of society as a whole and strengthening that of the health system in preventing and responding to sexual violence from a rights-based perspective" (WHO, 2016, p. 8) and

> addressing the root causes of sexual violence, such as gender inequality and sociocultural norms that tolerate violence, by empowering women and young people and ensuring access to comprehensive sexuality education, and combating negative male gender roles and stereotypical images of masculinity linked to the use of violence and a lack of respect for human rights.
>
> (WHO, 2016, p. 8)

In this, we see that sexual health can only be fulfilled through the adaptation of a broad set of sexual rights. In this view, sexual health comes to see the body of the individual as the locus of sexual rights and empowerment, yet also the site for potential sexualized violence. Moreover, education is seen as key in order to ensure that sexual rights are disseminated and picked up in the population while also ensuring that this education will lead to a more robust understanding of sexual norms and thus limit sexualized violence through combating what has been called "toxic masculinity" (Kupers, 2005). In the WHO action plan, the subject positions that are being created if we see it through the lens of "what is the problem represented to be?" can be divided into the following subject positions: (i) women and young people, who through education and knowledge will be empowered, and (ii) men who are in need of education in order to combat negative gender roles which will lead men to become the potential perpetrators of gender-based violence. While this in and of itself is laudable, it does beg the question of how to empower young boys and men in order to change their behavior. Moreover, while the strategy calls for calling out the "root cause" of sexual violence, larger structural factors beyond cultural norms seem to recede into the background. Education becomes a catchall for change, it seems, and while education is crucial, it is not easy to see or even read into the strategy what this education should include. It also seems to postulate that there is *one* ideal educational strategy to reach this goal, while less attention is paid to the local contexts in which these forms of strategies are to be implemented. Conversely, it also seems to state that there is such as thing as a "negative male gender role" across nations and cultures; thus, this subject position seems to become what Bowker and Star have called a "boundary object" (Bowker & Star, 2000; Leigh Star, 2010). While we agree that there is such a thing as a "negative male gender role," it is less clear what this gender role is across diverse countries and cultures. Research on masculinity and gender roles is a diverse field, and much attention has been accorded the issue of negative traits or gender role understanding amongst men (Connell, 1998, 2005; Kimmel, 2017; Kimmel et al., 2004). The tensions here are, of course, not new: these illustrate how rights perspectives come into contact with the dilemmas between universal and particular rights, an aspect which has haunted human rights research for a long time. In the case of sexual rights, the Norwegian strategy actually touches upon this when it deals with immigrants and asylum seekers coming to Norway. The strategy states that

> The right to decide over one's own body and good sexual health encompasses all human beings. Some young and adult people who have recently arrived in Norway from other countries already possess good knowledge around this topic while others lack knowledge on this topic. Education about sexuality and sexual health is included in a mandatory information plan for people living in immigration transit housing.
>
> (Ministry of Health and Social Services Norway, 2017, p. 20)

In this view, people from outside of Norway are perceived to either possess a form of knowledge that is "good" and in line with the knowledge and values highlighted in Norway or as lacking this and thus in need of a supplement, in this case, education, in order to make the Other fall in line with the knowledge regime of sexuality and sexual health in Norway.

LGBTQI communities and people living with HIV are often highlighted as being protected by the concept of sexual rights, as are the young and women in particular. In the strategies we have analyzed, this is clearly highlighted as being part of what sexual rights mean. LGBTQI rights are often defined in the material as being in need of protection *from* something or *someone*. In the case of Norway, we can read that

> In many cases, sexual freedom and sexual rights challenge traditional gender roles and are perceived by some as a threat to culture and values. Although attitudes towards gays have undergone a positive change, it can still be very difficult to be gay in ethnic and national minorities.
>
> (Ministry of Health and Social Services Norway, 2017, p. 25)

In this case, sexual rights are accorded importance in their capacity to provide protection from discrimination and stigma from other groups, in this case, ethnic and national minorities. Part of the sexual rights framework is also embedded in juridical statutes. A case in point would be the Irish strategy. In the Irish strategy, it is noted that "In 2010, the Civil Partnerships Act granted extensive rights and responsibilities to lesbian and gay couples that were previously only available to married couples. By June 2014, a total of 1,467 civil partnerships had taken place in Ireland" (An Roinn Siainte, 2015, p. 27). While the extension of civil partnership rights to same-sex couples has been perceived as a crucial step towards equality and civil rights for LGBTQI communities, it has also received criticism from within the same communities. Part of the criticism has not so much been the extension of the *right to marry* but more the need to "emulate heteronormative standards of partnership and family" (Duggan, 2002; Santos, 2013). Heteronormativity can be defined as "the assumption that heterosexuality is the default, preferred, 'normal' state for human beings because of the belief that people fall into one or other category of a strict gender binary" (Harris & White, 2018). Homonormativity, on the other hand, can thus be defined as "a politics that does not contest dominant heteronormativity assumptions and institutions but upholds and sustains them while promising the possibility of a demobilised gay culture anchored in domesticity and consumption" (Duggan, 2002, p. 50). Sexual rights when coupled with civil rights demonstrate a tension within the lexicon of sexual health: on the one hand, they are a boon in that they ensure equal rights and protection to LGBTQI communities. Yet, on the other hand, scholars such as Lisa Duggan (2002), David Halperin (2012), and Gayle Rubin (2011) have all noted the tensions embedded within this matrix. For one, the main criticism is that LGBTQI communities are accorded these sexual rights only within an already-existing framework of heterosexual family constellations. Here the right to live together and get married is predicated upon the heterosexual couple as the model for sexual and intimate lives. Moreover, it does not contest the institution of marriage as much as it emulates it. While our main contention is not to dispute or support either side of these claims, we do want to note that sexual rights as part of sexual health are predicated upon normative injunctions of how to live together and what rights should be accorded when people do so. This leads us to the final section of the chapter, which is a brief analysis of the many silences and areas *not mentioned* in these strategies. For Foucault and Bacchi, silence is not the absolute limit of discourse but rather spaces wherein we can learn and extract information about the things left unsaid, in this case, about what sexual health can be in the SDG era.

Incitement to discourse: sexual health and its silences

In the previous, we have argued that "sexual health" as a combination term affords governments various entry points into the government of people and different problems, problems that go far beyond sexual health as a mere biomedical problem. Sexual health can be said to encompass a broad array of what Epstein and Mamo have called "social niches" (2017). Yet while we agree with this statement and to a large degree are supportive of this, the strategies that we have looked at focus to a large degree on biomedical issues such as limiting and reducing STIs and HIV, reducing and preventing unwanted pregnancies, and aiding with sexual dysfunction through pharmaceutical interventions. Sexual rights are also very dominant, even more so in the Scandinavian framework than in the others.

In Chapter 3, we saw how the concept of sexual health has emerged through different position papers, reports, and strategies. One key claim there was that sexual health has to a large degree been dominated by precisely biomedical understandings of sexuality and health. Yet certain position papers have paid attention to the idea of pleasure and desire as being part of the holistic conceptualization of sexual health. In the strategies we have analyzed, the concept of pleasure seems to be all but absent.

A striking example of the near-absolute absence of pleasure as part of sexual health can be found by searching the strategies and reports that we have analyzed for the very word "pleasure." In doing this, we find the term is all but absent. In the WHO European strategy, the term is not even mentioned. In the strategy published by the Department of Health in England, the term is noted *once*: "Attitudes, for example the belief that condom use or male sterilization can decrease sexual pleasure, or the common misconception that all hormonal contraceptives lead to weight gain" (Department of Health, England, 2013). In the Irish case, pleasure is noted in the definition of sexuality, "Sexuality is a central aspect of being human and encompasses sex, gender identities and roles, sexual orientation, eroticism, pleasure, intimacy and reproduction" (An Roinn Siainte, 2015), and yet is never mentioned afterward. In the Norwegian case, pleasure is mentioned once directly but only passively as part of a broader focus on mental health issues which can *affect pleasure* (Ministry of Health and Social Services Norway, 2017). It is alluded to in the Foreword of Minister of Health Bent Høie through the usage of "a force," yet pleasure as such is never directly addressed in the strategy.

This silence is a telling silence of modern conceptions of sexual health within policy and health care. While pleasure is common in sexual health when it is defined in the public press and various self-help sources, both in press and online, as Epstein and Mamo note (2017), it is all but absent in public policy and biomedical conceptions of sexual health. Pleasure as part of sexual health seems to have vanished from the view of policy and politics; it is nowhere to be found in these strategies, even though sexual health clearly is also about pleasure. In the policy documents analyzed, sexual health can, perhaps a bit schematically, be reduced to (i) biomedical mechanisms pertaining to the body (sexual dysfunction, unwanted pregnancies), (ii) protecting the body from harm stemming from microbes (STIs and HIV), (iii) protecting the body from harm from other humans (sexual violence, discrimination, and stigma), and (iv) securing the body through legal and normative frameworks (sexual rights). Pleasure, on the other hand, is omitted as part of this. Michel Foucault noted in his work on the history of sexuality that a divide was ushered in in the 19th century between what he calls *ars erotica* and *scientia sexualis* (1990a). Foucault famously links this spilt to the emergence of what he called "the normalizing sciences": demography, psychology, medicine, and statistics. If the ancient Greeks possessed what he called an *ars erotica*, then "we," the moderns, have replaced that with *scientia sexualis* (Foucault, 1990a, p. 71). In the regime of *scientia sexualis*, based on modern medicine and psychology, sex (and, logically, pleasure) was seen as a *problem to be solved* (Foucault, 1990a, pp. 65–75). Sex within the logic of *scientia sexualis* was seen as something dangerous: pleasure, and in particular those pleasures deemed perverse, could be a threat not just to the person but indeed to society as a whole.

Sex and pleasure became objects of scientific knowledge that needed to be dissected and *known* through scientific methods in order to safeguard not just individuals but indeed the entire population. Sex and pleasure were thus put under a new regime of truth (Foucault, 1990a, pp. 68–69). In the policy documents we have analyzed, this seems to clearly be the case: sexual health in official public policy is highlighted contingent upon a biomedical regime of knowledge, supplemented with a legal and rights-based set of norms. Sexual health in these strategies is knowable, governable, and visible through regimes meant to tell the truth about different aspects of human health and sexuality. Yet pleasure is, as stated, omitted from this discourse.

Kane Race, writing in a related setting, touches upon this paradox relating to HIV research:

> Biomedical research and preventive efforts on HIV have often had a tendency to disregard sex as anything other than a confounding variable or complicating factor, within research and preventive campaigns thus our capacity to grasp it as a source of knowledge or scene of productively disorganizing intensity is diminished.
>
> (2016, p. 7)

The aversion to sex and pleasure seen in early HIV prevention efforts and to some extent present even today entails a paradox:

> The very expertise we might hope to cultivate for HIV prevention – expertise in sex as a form of praxis, a source of pedagogy, and potentially motivating encounter – is dissuaded if not actively undermined by some of the epistemic and professional frames that prominently organize responses to HIV.
>
> (Race, 2016, p. 9)

Within research on HIV prevention, pleasure and sex are often reduced to questions concerning clinical control.

> Did trial participants adhere to the dosing requirements? Are they telling the truth? How should we measure discrepancies? . . . Any interest or insight that research scientists or trial practitioners may have had into the sexual or everyday lives of trial participants was carefully excluded from consideration by the conventions that shape the discussion in such forums.
>
> (Race, 2016, p. 9)

This paradox can probably be extrapolated to a broad range of issues within sexual health: pleasure and sex are, in the previous strategies, seen as *problems to be overcome and not as sources of pedagogy or motivation.* The proof of this must be the overwhelming silence in relation to the very term "pleasure." Sexual health in the previous is firmly rooted in a regime of *scientia sexualis*, a regime where the truth about human sexuality and health can only be discerned through different forms of objective sciences.

Ars erotica, on the other hand, entailed in Foucault's rendition a form of knowledge of sensual pleasure. The knowledge and truth that this form of practice contained was a truth about pleasure itself: how pleasure could be experienced, intensified, or maximized (Foucault, 1990b). Finally, Foucault notes that this form of knowledge did not ask the question of what pleasures were permitted and which were forbidden: only the question of the pleasures themselves (1990b, pp. 30–31).

In the strategies and reports we have analyzed, pleasure as an object itself is never mentioned. In fact, it is rarely even mentioned. Phrases such as "well-being" and "health" are common, yet pleasure as part of sexual health is omitted. Pleasure seem to have been relegated to the margins when it comes to sexual health, and yet pleasure is, of course, the main driving force of human sexuality. Mamo and Epstein note that sexual health's meteoric rise in the lexicon of human health might also have been part of a implicit rhetorical move which has "sanitized sex" through linking sex to health and human rights (2017). Sexual health in the SDG era clearly seems to posit human sexuality and health as objects of science rather than arts. Moreover, sexual health in the SDG era is predicated upon a series of biomedical regimes of science which *extract* knowledge from the subject and the population as a whole.

It is worth noting here that the Greek word *eros* denotes sexual love, desire, and pleasure.[6] As such, we could dichotomize and say that *eros* refers to sex as a sensual matter, whereas *sexualis* refers to sex as an abstract concept, often coupled with the various sciences that have taken it as an object of study.

In the strategies that we have analyzed, sexual health is an object of science and of rights, of biomedicine and psychology. Love, desire, and pleasure are all but absent, and what has taken their place is health, well-being, and rights. While we are not intrinsically against this, there is something rather perplexing about sexual health strategies which so clearly avoid these terms. On a pedagogical note, the strategies highlight the ways in which young people should learn about reproductive rights, birth control, STI prevention, and sexual rights. *Eros* as a pedagogy of pleasure, on the other hand, is not to be found. Pleasure as part of sexual health seems to have been purified and sanitized through biomedical language and rights-based perspectives.

Sexual health in the post-SDG era seems to have embraced metrics, indicators, rights, and health as a way of talking about sex in relation to human health. It allows for the government of populations in the name of "healthy sexual health" and entangled with a rights perspective. Yet, might we not here also pause and wonder why pleasure, a cornerstone of sexuality, is left so silent in all the strategies that we have analyzed? One answer might be that pleasure is seen as belonging to the dominion of the private, yet this cannot explain everything: after all, so too do many of the other aspects that are included under the term "sexual health." Another possible explanation might be that pleasure is hard to quantify: in the SDG era, as we have seen, metrics and indicators have come to dominate the ways in which we govern health, including sexual health. Metrics offer an alleged way of objectively, effectively, and sustainably governing health. However, by omitting pleasure as part of sexual health in official policies, we might ask: Is it sustainable to avoid talking about pleasure as part of a holistic paradigm of sexual health? Is it sustainable to suppress the question of pleasure when we are dealing with sexual health policies?

In conclusion, and without offering an answer to these questions, we might problematize why pleasure has come to be shunned or suppressed in public policies that deal with sexual health. In the long run, it might not be sustainable to avoid the question of pleasure. Pleasure might be hard to standardize, to quantify and measure, yet it is undoubtedly a part of human sexuality and as such should be part of a sexual health regime that professes to be holistic and sustainable.

Notes

1 See Clive Barnett's article on the issue of problematization. https://nonsite.org/article/on-problematization
2 Ora Quick. www.oraquick.com/
3 See the DoD's webpage for the full transcript. http://archive.defense.gov/Transcripts/Transcript.aspx?TranscriptID=2636
4 For a small sample of research papers that call for more attention to the phenomena of chemsex and gay male sexuality, HIV, and STIs, see, for instance: Ahmed et al., 2016; Bourne et al., 2015; Hegazi et al., 2017; Ma & Perera, 2016; McCall et al., 2015; Pufall et al., 2016; Sewell et al., 2017; Weatherburn et al., 2017.
5 See the BMJ Blogspot for more information. https://blogs.bmj.com/sti/2018/05/04/heterosexual-chemsex/
6 See Merriam-Webster online dictionary. www.merriam-webster.com/dictionary/Eros

References

Abraham, J. (2010). Pharmaceuticalization of society in context: Theoretical, empirical and health dimensions. *Sociology, 44*(4), 603–622.

Ahmed, A. K., Weatherburn, P., Reid, D., Hickson, F., Torres-Rueda, S., Steinberg, P., & Bourne, A. (2016). Social norms related to combining drugs and sex ("chemsex") among gay men in South London. *International Journal of Drug Policy, 38*, 29–35.

An Roinn Siainte. (2015). *National sexual health strategy 2015–2020*. Department of Health. https://assets.gov.ie/7562/e5a5ac26eb22405aaf6538656564690a.pdf

Bacchi, C. (2000). Policy as discourse: What does it mean? Where does it get us? *Discourse: Studies in the Cultural Politics of Education, 21*(1), 45–57.

Bacchi, C. (2009). *Analysing policy*. Pearson Higher Education.

Bacchi, C. (2012). Why study problematizations? Making politics visible. *Open Journal of Political Science, 2*(1), 1.

Bacchi, C. (2015). The turn to problematization: Political implications of contrasting interpretive and poststructural adaptations. *Open Journal of Political Science, 5*.

Bacchi, C., & Goodwin, S. (2016). *Poststructural policy analysis: A guide to practice*. Springer.

Banda, J. (2015). Rapid home HIV testing: Risk and the moral imperatives of biological citizenship. *Body & Society, 21*(4), 24–47.

Bell, S. E., & Figert, A. E. (2012). Medicalization and pharmaceuticalization at the intersections: Looking backward, sideways and forward. *Social Science & Medicine, 75*(5), 775–783.

Biehl, J. (2007). Pharmaceuticalization: AIDS treatment and global health politics. *Anthropological Quarterly*, 1083–1126.

Bourne, A., Reid, D., Hickson, F., Torres-Rueda, S., & Weatherburn, P. (2015). Illicit drug use in sexual settings ("chemsex") and HIV/STI transmission risk behaviour among gay men in South London: Findings from a qualitative study. *Sexually Transmitted Infections, 91*(8), 564–568.

Bowker, G. C., & Star, S. L. (2000). *Sorting things out: Classification and its consequences*. MIT Press.

Choko, A. T., Desmond, N., Webb, E. L., Chavula, K., Napierala-Mavedzenge, S., Gaydos, C. A., Makombe, S. D., Chunda, T., Squire, S. B., French, N., Mwapasa, V., & Corbett, E. L. (2011). The uptake and accuracy of oral kits for HIV self-testing in high HIV prevalence setting: A cross-sectional feasibility study in Blantyre, Malawi. *PLoS Medicine, 8*(10), e1001102.

Clarke, A. E., Shim, J. K., Mamo, L., Fosket, J. R., & Fishman, J. R. (2010). Biomedicalization: Technoscientific transformations of health, illness, and US biomedicine. *Biomedicalization: Technoscience, Health, and Illness in the US*, 47–87.

Connell, R. W. (1998). Masculinities and globalization. *Men and Masculinities, 1*(1), 3–23.

Connell, R. W. (2005). *Masculinities*. Polity.

Department of Health, England. (2013). *A framework for sexual health improvement in England*. https://assets.publishing.service.gov.uk/government/uploads/system/uploads/attachment_data/file/142592/9287-2900714-TSO-SexualHealthPolicyNW_ACCESSIBLE.pdf

Duggan, L. (2002). The new homonormativity: The sexual politics of neoliberalism. *Materializing Democracy: Toward a Revitalized Cultural Politics*, 175–194.

Epstein, S. (1995). The construction of lay expertise: AIDS activism and the forging of credibility in the reform of clinical trials. *Science, Technology, & Human Values, 20*(4), 408–437.

Epstein, S. (1996). *Impure science: AIDS, activism, and the politics of knowledge* (vol. 7). University of California Press.

Epstein, S. (2003). An incitement to discourse: Sociology and the history of sexuality. *Sociological Forum, 18*(3).

Epstein, S., & Mamo, L. (2017). The proliferation of sexual health: Diverse social problems and the legitimation of sexuality. *Social Science & Medicine, 188*, 176–190.

Foucault, M. (1984). *The Foucault reader* (P. Rabinow, ed., p. 173). Pantheon Books.

Foucault, M. (1990a). *The history of sexuality: An introduction* (R. Hurley, trans., vol. I.). Vintage.

Foucault, M. (1990b). *The use of pleasure: Volume two of the history of sexuality* (R. Hurley, trans.). Vintage.

Foucault, M. (2001). *Fearless speech*. Semiotext(e).

Foucault, M. (2012). *The history of sexuality, vol. 2: The use of pleasure*. Vintage.

Foucault, M., Lotringer, S., & Hochroth, L. (2007). *The politics of truth*. MIT Press.

Giami, A. (2002). Sexual health: The emergence, development, and diversity of a concept. *Annual Review of Sex Research, 13*(1), 1–35.

Giddens, A. (2013). *The consequences of modernity*. John Wiley & Sons.

Hakim, J. (2017). *Chemsex: Anatomy of a sex panic*. Rowman & Littlefield.

Halperin, D. M. (2012). *How to be gay*. Harvard University Press.

Harris, J., & White, V. (2018). *A dictionary of social work and social care*. Oxford University Press.

Hegazi, A., Lee, M., Whittaker, W., Green, S., Simms, R., Cutts, R., Nagington, M., Nathan, B., & Pakianathan, M. (2017). Chemsex and the city: Sexualised substance use in gay bisexual and other men who have sex with men attending sexual health clinics. *International Journal of STD & AIDS, 28*(4), 362–366.

Jantarapakde, J., Himmad, K., Sungsing, T., Anand, T., Nitpolprasert, C., Promthong, S., Waiwinya, W., Meekrua, P., Sukthongsa, S., Hongwiangchan, S., Upanun, N., Trachunthong, D., Barisi, S., Jirajariyavej, S., Charoenying, S., Mills, S., Vannakit,

R., Cowing, M., Buchbinder, S., & Hongwiangchan, S. (2018). *Online supervised HIV self-testing identified high HIV yield among Thai men who have sex with men and transgender women.* Paper presented at the *Journal of the International AIDS Society.*

Kenworthy, N., Thomann, M., & Parker, R. (2018). From a global crisis to the "end of AIDS": New epidemics of signification. *Global Public Health, 13*(8), 960–971.

Kimmel, M. S. (2017). *Angry white men: American masculinity at the end of an era.* Hachette.

Kimmel, M. S., Hearn, J., & Connell, R. W. (2004). *Handbook of studies on men and masculinities.* Sage Publications.

Kupers, T. A. (2005). Toxic masculinity as a barrier to mental health treatment in prison. *Journal of Clinical Psychology, 61*(6), 713–724.

Leigh Star, S. (2010). This is not a boundary object: Reflections on the origin of a concept. *Science, Technology, & Human Values, 35*(5), 601–617.

Lovelock, M. (2018). Sex, death and austerity: Resurgent homophobia in the British tabloid press. *Critical Studies in Media Communication,* 1–15.

Lupton, D. (2012). M-health and health promotion: The digital cyborg and surveillance society. *Social Theory & Health, 10*(3), 229–244.

Lupton, D. (2013a). The digitally engaged patient: Self-monitoring and self-care in the digital health era. *Social Theory & Health, 11*(3), 256–270.

Lupton, D. (2013b). Quantifying the body: Monitoring and measuring health in the age of mHealth technologies. *Critical Public Health, 23*(4), 393–403.

Lupton, D. (2015). Quantified sex: A critical analysis of sexual and reproductive self-tracking using apps. *Culture, Health & Sexuality, 17*(4), 440–453.

Ma, R., & Perera, S. (2016). Safer "chemsex": GPs' role in harm reduction for emerging forms of recreational drug use. *British Journal of General Practice, 66.*

Mamo, L. (2003). *Sexuality, reproduction and biomedical negotiations: An analysis of achieving pregnancy in the absence of heterosexuality* (PhD dissertation). University of California.

McCall, H., Adams, N., Mason, D., & Willis, J. (2015). What is chemsex and why does it matter? *British Medical Journal, 351.*

Meneu, R. (2018). Life medicalization and the recent appearance of "pharmaceuticalization". *Farmacia Hospitalaria: Organo Oficial de Expresion Científica de la Sociedad Espanola de Farmacia Hospitalaria, 42*(4), 174–179.

Miller, P., & Rose, N. (2017). Political power beyond the state: Problematics of government. In *Foucault and law* (pp. 191–224). Routledge.

Ministry of Health and Social Services Norway. (2017). *Snakk om det! Strategi for seksuell helse 2017–2022.* https://www.regjeringen.no/contentassets/284e09615fd04338a817e1 160f4b10a7/strategi_seksuell_helse.pdf

Ministry of Solidarity and Health France. (2017). *National sexual health strategy.* Government of France.

Osborne, T. (1997). Of health and statecraft. *Foucault, Health and Medicine,* 173–188.

Public Health England. (2015). *Health promotion for sexual and reproductive health and HIV.* https://assets.publishing.service.gov.uk/government/uploads/system/uploads/ attachment_data/file/488090/SRHandHIVStrategicPlan_211215.pdf

Pufall, E., Kall, M., Shahmanesh, M., Nardone, A., Gilson, R., & Delpech, V. (2016). *Chemsex and high-risk sexual behaviours in HIV-positive men who have sex with men.* Paper presented at the Conference on retroviruses and opportunistic infections. https:// www.iapac.org/files/2019/10/FTC2019-Labayen-de-Inza.pdf

Rabinow, P. (1984). Polemics, politics, and problematizations: An interview with Michel Foucault. *The Foucault Reader*, 380–390.

Race, K. (2016). Reluctant objects: Sexual pleasure as a problem for HIV biomedical prevention. *GLQ: A Journal of Lesbian and Gay Studies, 22*(1), 1–31.

Rubin, G. (2011). *Deviations: A Gayle Rubin reader*. Duke University Press.

Sandset, T. (2019). "HIV both starts and stops with me": Configuring the neoliberal sexual actor in HIV prevention. *Sexuality & Culture*, 1–17.

Santos, A. C. (2013). Are we there yet? Queer sexual encounters, legal recognition and homonormativity. *Journal of Gender Studies, 22*(1), 54–64.

Sewell, J., Miltz, A., Lampe, F. C., Cambiano, V., Speakman, A., Phillips, A. N., Stuart, D., Gilson, R., Asboe, D., Clarke, A., Collins, S., Hart, G., Elford, J., Rodger, A. J., & Nwokolo, N. (2017). Poly drug use, chemsex drug use, and associations with sexual risk behaviour in HIV-negative men who have sex with men attending sexual health clinics. *International Journal of Drug Policy, 43*, 33–43.

Shammas, V. L., & Sandset, T. J. (2020). *Reproduction and the welfare state: Notes on Norwegian biopolitics*. Oslo Metropolitan University.

Sunhedsstyrelsen. (2018). *Seksuel sunhed*. https://www.sst.dk/da/viden/seksuel-sundhed

UNAIDS. (2014). *90-90-90: An ambitious treatment target to help end the AIDS epidemic*. UNAIDS.

UNAIDS. (2017). *Ending AIDS: Progress towards the 90-90-90 targets. Global AIDS update*. UNAIDS.

UNAIDS. (2019). *Global AIDS monitoring 2019: Indicators for the monitoring of the 2016 political declaration on ending AIDS 208*. https://indicatorregistry.unaids.org/sites/default/files/2019-global-aids-monitoring_en_0.pdf

United Nations General Assembly (UN) (2015). *Transforming our world: the 2030 agenda for sustainable development*. Division for Sustainable Development Goals.

Walensky, R. P., & Paltiel, A. D. (2006). Rapid HIV testing at home: Does it solve a problem or create one? *Annals of Internal Medicine, 145*(6), 459–462.

Weatherburn, P., Hickson, F., Reid, D., Torres-Rueda, S., & Bourne, A. (2017). Motivations and values associated with combining sex and illicit drugs ("chemsex") among gay men in South London: Findings from a qualitative study. *Sexually Transmitted Infections, 93*(3), 203–206.

WHO. (2002). *Defining sexual health: Report of a technical consultation on sexual health*. WHO.

WHO. (2016). *Action plan for sexual and reproductive health: Towards achieving the 2030 agenda for sustainable development in Europe – leaving no one behind*. WHO.

6   Controlling AIDS
The 90–90–90 targets and the politics of counting

Introduction

In the SDG era, the rise of indicators, metrics, and data-driven health governance has taken center stage. Indeed, the SDGs themselves are predicated in many cases upon the entanglements between aspirational goal setting, indicator-driven targets, and the collection of data. Sexual health as such is no exemption from this. In the following, we will examine the case of how data, indicators, and metrics impact and structure efforts to control and "end" the HIV epidemic. HIV has a privileged position in the sphere of sexual health. It is little wonder that this book has also dedicated a rather large section to how the HIV efforts in the SDG era are unfolding. A very large part of that process has been through the scale-up and rollout of targeted interventions and subsequently metrics and indicator-driven efforts to "end AIDS."

We want in the following to focus on this process and the mechanisms of these issues to link the emerging indicator-driven HIV effort with the ideology of sustainability. In the SDGs themselves, HIV is, as mentioned before, listed in Target 3.3, which states, "By 2030, end the epidemics of AIDS." The listed indicator for this is Indicator 3.3.1 which is "number of new HIV infections per 1,000 uninfected population, by sex, age and key populations" (Resolution, 2015). The target and the indicator are linked through a form of logic that states that in order to reach the target, we need to monitor the indicator while at the same time working towards the target goal. However, the SDGs say very little about the *methods* of reaching the target, and the SDGs do not say anything about the ways in which we are to lower the indicated denominator mentioned in the indicator. In the case of SDG 3.3.1, the SDGs do not mention any specific method for lowering the number of new HIV infections. As such, several methods for lowering rates of new HIV infections have been proposed historically, yet none more prominently, perhaps, than the current 90–90–90 model proposed by UNAIDS.

The 90–90–90 targets state that by 2020, 90% of all people living with HIV will know their HIV status, that 90% of all people with diagnosed HIV infection will receive sustained antiretroviral therapy, and that 90% of all people receiving antiretroviral therapy will have achieved viral load suppression (UNAIDS, 2014). This chapter seeks to explore how the 90–90–90 targets as a method and model for reaching the SDG target of "ending AIDS" by 2030, as well as a method which can be linked to Indicator 3.3.1, contain within themselves several potential pitfalls. These potential pitfalls are linked to some of the normative effects that follow in the wake of the targets but also some of the more central debates around what sustainability is and how the very nature of sustainability becomes entangled with discourses of cost-effectiveness as well as the quantification of targets and goals. A brief historical background of the current response to the global HIV/AIDS epidemic is needed.

Sustainability in the HIV discourse

The HIV/AIDS epidemic is the only epidemic to have been taken up in the UN Security Council twice, with two subsequent UN resolutions, Res. 1983 and Res. 1308.[1] In both cases, the HIV/AIDS epidemic was framed as a crisis of global proportions, such as in Res. 1308, where the Security Council stated: "the HIV/AIDS pandemic, if unchecked, may pose a risk to stability and security."[2] This was reiterated in Res.1983, when the Security Council made the statement that "HIV poses one of the most formidable challenges to the development, progress, and stability of societies and requires an exceptional and comprehensive global response."[3] Kenworthy et al. state that

> if the decade following the first Durban AIDS Conference in 2000 was marked by discourses about an epidemic "out of control" and a politics of emergency that justified exceptional activism and action, the decade of AIDS responses beginning in 2010 has been distinctly framed by declarations that an AIDS-free generation is within our grasp.
>
> (Kenworthy et al., 2018, p. 960)

The so-called ARV era ushered in what has been called "a period of optimism."[4] However, the HIV epidemic was by the late 1990s and early 2000s framed as a "global crisis" and in particular an African crisis (Piot, 2003; Sibanda, 2000). The *New Scientist* reported in November of 2003 that the UN sounded the alarms and that 2003 had "the highest ever number of new HIV infections and deaths around the world."[5] Then-UNAIDS Executive Director Peter Piot stated, "It is quite clear that our current global efforts remain entirely inadequate for an epidemic that is continuing to spiral out of control."[6] Jack Chow, assistant director-general for HIV/AIDS, TB, and malaria at the World Health Organization, added, "In two short decades HIV/AIDS has tragically become the premier disease of mass destruction."[7] We should note that a few years after 2003, the financial crisis of 2007–2008 heralded a shift in funding which also spurred the need for a new way of conceptualizing the HIV epidemic. Kenworthy et al. state that "as a result of the financial crisis, a series of important donor withdrawals marked the beginning of a shift from 'scale-up' to 'scale-down' that still is visible today" (2018, p. 962), wherein donors are asking recipients to do more with less and "optimize" their HIV treatment and prevention programs. This also meant that a new discourse of sustainability, accountability, and country ownership, as well as the much-talked-about the paradigm of transitioning from donor funding to domestic funding, took form as a way for donor countries to avoid long-term treatment commitments as well as resource-intensive programs. Following the scale-down and the paradigm of doing more with less, various national agencies and donor organizations shifted their funding strategies from general population and treatment scale-ups onto new targets such as "key populations" and investments in biomedical prevention technologies and techniques.

90–90–90: three metrics as a transformative agenda?

One of current cornerstones in the global HIV effort has been the so-called 90–90–90 targets. The 90–90–90 targets were born out of a realization that people living with HIV who reached "undetectable viral load numbers" were living close to normal life expectancies and were unable to transmit HIV onwards. This has been called "treatment as prevention," as it is both treatment for people living with HIV as well as serving as a preventive technology in limiting HIV transmission.

Guillaume Lachenal states that "TasP [treatment as prevention] began as an exercise in epidemiological modeling" which tried to answer the question of "Knowing that antiretroviral therapy (ART) drastically reduces HIV transmission, what population-level effect would result from screening and immediately treating all HIV-infected individuals?" (Lachenal, 2013, p. 70). This realization also points us to the influence of modeling and models within the current drive towards reaching the SDGs, what Rhodes et al. call "the model society" (Rhodes & Lancaster, 2020; Rhodes et al., 2020). Once it became clear that *treatment was also prevention*, modeling exercises were conducted to forecast what effects widespread treatment might have not only for the quality of life and life expectancies for people living with HIV but also for rates of new cases of HIV infections.

The optimism that the models of the 90–90–90 targets brought can be seen in, for example, the new discourse of UNAIDS.

In 2014, then-UNAIDS Executive Director Michel Sidibé took to the stage in Hanoi at a UNAIDS summit and stated that

> This bold new set of targets, 90–90–90, will do more than reduce new HIV infections and AIDS-related deaths. It will be a transformative agenda for reaching people who are left behind. . . . 90–90–90 is our path to victory. It is our path to the end of this epidemic worldwide. When we talk about ending AIDS, we mean that by 2030, HIV and AIDS will no longer threaten human life. Of course, there will be new cases of HIV, but the virus will no longer be a public health danger.[8]

This quote from the launch of the 90–90–90 targets in 2014 points to perhaps the most important pillar in the work towards the end of AIDS, that is, the roll-out and scale-up of global "test, treat and retain" efforts operationalized and quantified through the metrics of 90–90–90. This set into motion a broad push amongst nations and cities to be the first to reach these targets. As a response to this, UNAIDS releases data on the progress towards the 90–90–90 targets and which countries have either reached them, are close to reaching them, or are "lagging behind." Three years later, in 2017, for instance, UNAIDS stated that seven countries had achieved 90–90–90. These were Botswana, Cambodia, Denmark, Iceland, Singapore, Sweden, and the United Kingdom (UNAIDS, 2017, p. 31). In connection to the report *Ending AIDS. Progress Towards the 90–90–90 Targets* (UNAIDS, 2017), then-Executive Director Michel Sidibé stated that

> When I launched the 90–90–90 targets three years ago, many people thought they were impossible to reach. Today, the story is very different. Families, communities, cities, and countries have witnessed a transformation, with access to HIV treatment accelerating in the past three years. A record 19.5 million people are accessing antiretroviral therapy, and for the first time, more than half of all people living with HIV are on treatment. . . . Global solidarity and shared responsibility have driven the success we have achieved so far. This must be sustained. . . . I remain optimistic. This report demonstrates the power of the 90–90–90 targets and what can be achieved in a short time.
>
> (UNAIDS, 2017, p. 6)

Clearly, in both 2014 and 2017, UNAIDS and the world saw the potential in the 90–90–90 targets as a way of "ending AIDS." In working with these targets, one might get the sense that the end of AIDS will come when we have reached the 90–90–90 targets. The slogan, as well as the subsequent target setting, might give us the impression that the end of AIDS is some sort of final event, or that once the targets have been reached, the end has come. However, since the 90–90–90 targets are about epidemic control, continual work is needed to maintain the numbers. The slogan of ending AIDS and the 90–90–90 targets with its set deadlines belie the fact that ending AIDS through these targets is not a static and "one-off" event. Without a vaccine or a cure, the end of AIDS will need to be *maintained*, and this will require continual monitoring, progress reporting, and most of all, continual engagement from all stakeholders. This is also problematic in terms of the SDGs: the SDGs themselves seem to postulate that if we work towards all the targets and reach them in 2030, we somehow will have "reached" the SDGs. Yet many, if not most, of the SDG targets are of such a nature that there must be a *continual process of maintaining progress*. The SDG 2030 deadline seems from this perspective both simplistic and even naïve, as there cannot be a final event which is the achievement of the SDGs. In the case of HIV as part of the SDGs, "ending AIDS" surely is a continual process that needs to be maintained.

This aspect could be seen, as Sara Davis shows us, when, in 2019, UNAIDS launched its *Miles to Go* report (UNAIDS, 2018). This time, updated data showed that the list mentioned previously was reduced to six, and while Botswana and the United Kingdom were still on the list, the others from the 2016 list had fallen out (Davis, 2020). They, in turn, had been replaced by Eswatini, Namibia, and the Netherlands (UNAIDS, 2018, p. 72). *While the end of AIDS has come to sig-nify a new form of thinking about the HIV epidemic*, the notion that there will be an "event" that is the end of AIDS, a sort of punctuation mark of the HIV epidemic, should be tempered by a realization that epidemic control is not a result but indeed a state of continually maintaining control. As such, ending AIDS through the 90–90–90 targets and the notion of epidemic control is a continual process of maintaining control, both at the level of the nation-state and at the level of the individual. This in turn produces many of the tensions between evidence-based knowledge; global interests and goals; and local needs, values, and desires. Sustainability in this view is perhaps best seen as those interventions which produce the optimal form of epidemic control, and if this is the case, then sustainability is also about control: sustainability might then also have a more authoritative side to it than we might have realized. Sustainability in the HIV effort is about control as much as it is about empowerment, and as such, we should also pay attention to the various aspects of sustainability and control within the current HIV effort.

People and places: focusing on the "right places and the right people"

Ending AIDS as part of the SDGs and sustainability thinking was born at the intersection between novel biomedical pharmaceuticals, advanced epidemiological modeling studies, political tensions between donor and recipient countries, and a new economic reality in the wake of the financial crisis. With declining global funds dedicated to the HIV/AIDS efforts, donor countries and organizations started to talk more about the need for "strategic" interventions that would "maximize impact." This language was adopted by the President's Emergency Plan for AIDS Relief, in particular through the renewed plan to focus on thirteen countries that are near reaching "epidemic control."[9] PEPFAR has programs in fifty countries, yet with its new strategy of focusing on a select group of thirteen countries that are close to achieving epidemic control, efforts are being redirected to these thirteen countries. The countries are Botswana, Côte d'Ivoire, Haiti, Kenya, Lesotho, Malawi, Namibia, Rwanda, Swaziland, Tanzania, Uganda, Zambia, and Zimbabwe. Of note is the fact that all of them are sub-Saharan African countries, signaling what PEPFAR has called its "transitioning out" of many low-prevalence and middle-income countries in Eastern Europe, Central Asia, Asia, and Latin America and the Caribbean.

In the aftermath of the announcement that PEPFAR would shift its focus onto these thirteen countries, renowned online media outlet Devex ran a series of articles on the implications of this shift. In the series, it was noted that "some nonpriority countries have seen funds shrink" and that "dramatic cuts to two priority countries during the current funding round, Tanzania and Kenya, took civil society organizations by surprise."[10] Furthermore, it was noted that "with these cuts, PEPFAR is intensifying its message that if a country is not making progress toward specific targets, either for programmatic or policy reasons, then the money will go elsewhere."[11] Part of this was linked to how PEPFAR expected and expects recipient countries to "do their part"; that is, domestic funding dedicated to HIV efforts needs to be in line with targets set by PEPFAR. Furthermore, PEPFAR noted that it needed Kenya's delayed "population-based HIV impact assessment survey" to understand the state of Kenya's HIV epidemic. It also noted that a possible concern was the increasingly hostile environment emerging towards vulnerable populations in Tanzania, as well as "the country program's underperformance in some areas of its response."[12] Leveraging progress towards the 90–90–90 targets as well as concerns over human rights and economic responsibility, PEPFAR has been able to reorient its efforts towards the thirteen countries in its new strategy. This is also is done in the name of sustainability, as the thirteen priority countries are seen as scoring higher on the PEPFAR sustainability index.

This also highlights the well-known problem of global health partnerships, which is often analyzed as less partnership and more "clientism," and "global health diplomacy," wherein power is brokered through developmental and humanitarian aid (Adams et al., 2008; Feldman & Ticktin, 2010; Kenworthy, 2014; Kenworthy & Parker, 2014). It also sheds light on the power of the 90–90–90 targets as metrics that serve to divide recipient countries into those that are on the one hand "keeping the pace," those that "are on track," and, on the other hand, those that are "lagging behind" and "not keeping the pace." By utilizing progress towards epidemic control, PEPFAR can leverage power through threatening or even cutting funding to recipient countries. This also has consequences for how we perceive what is sustainable or not. If, as Engebretsen et al. claim, sustainability was in the early 1990s associated with the durability of a program rather than, as it is now, the ability to self-improve, (Engebretsen et al., 2016), then the ability to progress along the 90–90–90 continuum speaks of this new rationale for thinking about sustainability. "Keeping the pace" and "being on track" are considered being sustainable, while lagging behind and not being on track signify an unsustainable ability to self-improve along the quantifiable metric scale of the 90–90–90 targets. This shows how metrics such as the 90–90–90 targets become crucial for leveraging political power in the name of sustainability.

Monitoring progress and re-definitions of sustainability

A case in point would be South Africa. South Africa is not a priority country for PEPFAR, yet it has the largest HIV epidemic in the world and as such has received funds from PEPFAR. As an article in *Business Live* notes, South Africa received about $670m in fiscal year 2018.[13] Yet PEPFAR noted in a letter that "progress has been grossly sub-optimal and insufficient to reach epidemic control"; thus, PEPFAR would cut funding to 400 million dollars for fiscal year 2019.[14] The resulting tension can be seen in the outcry from activists in South Africa, who noted that patients in South Africa should not fall victim to the dysfunctions of the South African health system and that the cuts might undermine the HIV efforts in the country.[15] Here we see the conflicts between, on the one hand, PEPFAR's focus on sustainability through cost-effectiveness and reaching the 90–90–90 targets and, on the other hand, the South African government's priorities and own needs, as well as activists who decry the decision by stating that people living with HIV will become trapped between PEPFAR's decision to cut funds and the South African government's "dysfunctional" system.

By monitoring a range of metrics, among these the 90–90–90 targets, PEPFAR discerns what is sustainable or unsustainable. Yet it is people living with HIV in South Africa that are at risk of suffering from the inability of the health system to improve *and*, at the same time, PEPFAR's technocratic conceptualization of what is sustainable or not.

In an economic and political climate where programs are expected to "do more, with less," a renewed focus on targeting "the right people and the right places" has emerged.

The focus on strategic interventions that would yield maximum impact has meant that the language of cost-effectiveness has come to dominate the end-of-AIDS narrative. With the implementation of the 90–90–90 targets, the end of AIDS could be scaled to fit any location and any population; that is, subsets could be analyzed according to their progress along with the 90–90–90 targets, as well as any geographical unit, as long as the data was available. This has meant an increase in focus on data gathering as well as establishing data infrastructures that can collect and monitor progress. In turn, using epidemiological data in combination with various emerging mapping technologies means that health care authorities can produce so-called "heat maps" or "hot spots" to show where the epidemic is concentrated and then position clinics, hospitals, and outreach programs where they are most needed (Davis, 2020).

Sustainable epidemic control – quantifiable measures

This new shift in policy and in donor dynamics is also entangled with the language of sustainability. PEPFAR has not only launched a new strategic focus, as we have seen, but has done so through the implementation of what is called the "sustainability index and dashboard" (SID). The SID is a tool comprising ninety questions spread across fifteen elements which forty-one PEPFAR countries report on annually. PEPFAR states that

> PEPFAR has set out to measure for the first time where countries are situated on the sustainability spectrum, with the aim of providing new data to inform annual PEPFAR investments and an opportunity for a dedicated sustainability dialogue with national stakeholders.
>
> (PEPFAR, 2017, p. 1)

Sustainability in this setting refers to the ability of a country to domestically fund, manage, and monitor its HIV response. The SIDs offer a quantifiable manner of evaluating and monitoring PEPFAR recipient countries and their progress towards "sustainable epidemic control." This is done by quantifying the ninety questions across fifteen elements and then giving each of the fifteen elements a score from 0 to 10. On this scale, a score below 3.50 indicates unsustainable, which requires significant investment; 3.50–6.99 indicates emerging sustainability; 7.00–8.49 indicates approaching sustainability; and 8.50–10.00 indicates sustainable and requires no additional funding (PEPFAR, 2017, p. 1). The SIDs, however, are not only used to monitor the HIV landscape of each country in question; they are also used by PEPFAR to plan investments and strategies for donor planning. By quantifying sustainability, strategies and priority programs can be set up. However, this has also led to a new manner of rhetorically shifting funding priorities and goals. Since the underlying goal is that each country should more and more take over the HIV effort by domestic funding, countries that perform well on the SIDs are expected to receive less money from PEPFAR and bear a greater burden of the funding effort by providing more domestic funds.

While this sounds fair enough, using this metrics-based system also allows for a much more top-down and donor-driven process of reaching the end of AIDS. It also drives a wedge between those countries that perform well on the SID and those that do not. A case in point would be Kenya, which in 2018 received an 18% drop in funding mostly attributed to its performance on the SID and in 2020 was anticipated to receive even less funding.[16] Yet this does not mean that countries that perform poorly also receive more support; on the contrary. A case in point here would be South Africa and Nigeria, countries with large generalized epidemics. Both countries received warnings by PEPFAR that their performance had been sub-optimal and that they needed to ramp up progress on the SID to "unlock" further funding (Center for Policy Impact in Global Health, 2019).[17] Here sustainability, when quantified and translated from a concept to indicator-driven governance, clearly also becomes a tool for political leverage.

Sustainability – conceptual changes

If we see this through a conceptual history of the term "sustainability," we can clearly see a shift in not only HIV efforts globally but indeed in what the concept of sustainability now means. Engebretsen et al. have mapped the conceptual changes in what sustainability has meant in developmental aid discourses and health (2016). In so doing, they first note that "there has been a pronounced shift in the meaning of sustainability, to the extent that the current use of the term risks deflecting support away from the weakest to those who have the ability to self-improve" (Engebretsen et al., 2016, p. e225). PEPFAR's shift in focus and the deployment of the SID clearly reflect this form of logic: self-improvement through better scoring on the SID with the ultimate goal of "country ownership" is clearly aligned with the findings of Engebretsen et al. They also argue that the conceptual shift that we see in the use of the term "sustainability" is one that goes in three stages: in the early 1990s, sustainability is referred to as durability of a health care program, independent of how the finances were assured. In the late 1990s, sustainability is now thought of as the adaptation of Western values such as "good governance" and "democracy," while in the 2000s and onwards, sustainability is more and more defined as the recipients' determination and ability to self-improve (Engebretsen et al., 2016, p. e225). PEPFAR's SIDs and recent alignment with the 90–90–90 targets reflect this in many ways. Good governance and democracy are all part of the SIDs, yet more so, new technocratic values have also entered the discourse. To self-improve is also to be able to have the tools to monitor this improvement; thus, part of the SIDs and the 90–90–90 targets is also to have data-driven infrastructure, epidemiological, and health data access and a broad range of technological interventions. No longer is it enough to profess support for good governance or democracy, but now countries must also support a data-driven approach to HIV and other sexual health issues. In an almost uncanny parallel, we see many of the same shifts in the understanding of what sustainability is in PEPFAR by way of looking at the findings from Engebretsen et al. Once again they state that "in the *DAC Strategies for Sustainable Development* from 2001, sustainability was associated with 'continuous improvement' as well as with 'monitoring' and systems which are 'domestically driven'" (Engebretsen et al., 2016, p. e226). Looking through PEPFARs new strategies as well as the SID, sustainability refracted through PEPFAR's new focus clearly is also a focus on monitoring, domestically driven funding efforts, and country ownership. In a very real manner, the SID and the emphasis on sustainable epidemic control shows that with

> the ideal of continuous improvement incorporated in the current concept of sustainability comes new expectations of self-management and self-assistance. Rather than reducing interference from high-income countries and maximizing the freedom of the recipient country, this shift implies interfering in a new manner by imposing a new ideology of managing one's freedom in the right way.
>
> (Engebretsen et al., 2016, p. e226)

PEPFAR's new strategy of reaching sustainable epidemic control in alignment with the 90–90–90 targets thus produces a new form of governance within global health, one which focuses on freedom and ownership but in a highly specific manner. The danger with this is, of course, that several studies show that when PEPFAR shifts its donor priorities and strategies away from direct service provision to country ownership, vulnerable communities suffer the most. These studies show that "civil society organizations, which typically provide services for key populations, tend to be vulnerable during transitions to country ownership due to reduced funding, exclusion from the transition planning process, and lack of absorption into a government-owned response" (Center for Policy Impact in Global Health, 2019, p. 7). Sustainability when defined as the ability for self-improvement as criteria for funding also means, conceptually speaking, that we risk funding only those who have the ability or desire to self-improve along the lines chosen by Western powers through a narrow and often technocratic set of criteria. We can end this section with a word of caution from Engebretsen et al. which is just as apt for our analysis of PEPFAR's recent shift in priorities when they state that

> Using sustainability as a selection criterion risks privileging recipients who have the capacity to gain control over health and living conditions and

exclude others as unworthy needy. It would be a paradox if the emphasis on sustainability ended up in preventing global equity and justice instead of promoting it.

(Engebretsen et al., 2016, p. e226)

In the new end-of-AIDS narrative, as it has emerged through the language of the 90–90–90 targets, the focus on monitoring sub-populations and their progress along the 90–90–90 continuum is highlighted in several strategies. In a comment on the *Lancet-UNAIDS Commission*, Lo and Horton write that "our Commission calls for all aspects of a comprehensive AIDS response to be funded and *targeted* where they will make the most difference, either in *geographical hotspots* or among *populations most at risk* of HIV" (2015, p. 107, our italics). The same has been echoed by UNAIDS, which has called for "programs to focus on 'location and population'." Besides, PEPFAR has stated that "there is a 'need to do the right things in the right places at the right time'," and the Global Fund adds to this by saying, "there is a need to 'target resources to areas with the greatest need'."

The end of AIDS envisioned through the 90–90–90 targets thus opens up a very specific frame for talking about and implementing programs and interventions. These are often contingent upon data-driven epidemiology, cost-effectiveness models, and the notion that interventions need to be targeted. Sustainability in this view is less about a holistic concept and more predicated upon a technocratic system of cost-effectiveness and computational power. The human element is often lost, it seems, in the forecasting of models and economic calculations.

With the introduction of the "treatment as prevention" paradigm which the 90–90–90 targets build on, a new way of "tracking" the end of AIDS has come about. By quantifying these goals, the global response to the HIV epidemic has become more geared towards counting and measuring progress through numbers that respond to the 90–90–90 targets. Indeed, as the UNAIDS slogan goes; "the old saying 'What gets measured gets done' may be a cliché, but is still very true for the response to HIV."[18] In turning to the 90–90–90 targets, a new norm within the global effort to "bend the arc of the epidemic" was born. As UNAIDS states:

> the 90–90–90 targets have become a central pillar of the global quest to end the AIDS epidemic. The targets reflect a fundamental shift in the world's approach to HIV treatment, moving it away from a focus on the number of people accessing antiretroviral therapy and towards the importance of maximizing viral suppression among people living with HIV.

(UNAIDS, 2017, p. 8)

In this quote, the universal ambition and usefulness of the 90–90–90 targets are highlighted. Furthermore, the quote also highlights a new way of not only understanding how to best control and contain, even end, the AIDS epidemic, but also that these targets are "global" in their scope. Furthermore, this framing of the global utility of the 90–90–90 targets not only spatializes the implementation of these targets across the entire globe, but it also stipulates that the 90–90–90 targets become a global way of *counting* and *tracking* the *progress* of ending AIDS. The logic of tracking and counting through the 90–90–90 targets points to the importance given to the universality of metrics in global health and specifically in HIV/AIDS efforts. With the launch of the fast-track strategy, UNAIDS underlined the importance of numerical targets by stating that "targets drive progress," "targets promote accountability," and finally, that "targets underscore that ending the AIDS epidemic is achievable" (UNAIDS, 2014, p. 11). However, with these arguments about how sustainability has changed to a discourse of proving the ability for self-improvement, we might postulate that the use of metrics might not only promote accountability but risk individualizing each nation's *responsibility* rather than accountability. Moreover, accountability might not mean in this discourse a collaborative effort to end AIDS or control the HIV epidemic; rather, it might come to indicate a narrow discourse based on a logic of numerical *accounting* – that is, accountability comes to be solely defined as the ability to account for progress along the metrics provided, thus reducing accountability to a purely mathematical endeavor.

The notion that numerical targets promote accountability is particularly striking here. Since funding is scarce for the global HIV effort, numerical targets also act as disciplinary metrics. Agencies such as the Global Fund, UNAIDS, and local organizations that receive funds from, for instance, PEPFAR, need to show progress along the 90–90–90 cascade to argue both for success as well as replenishments of their funds from donors. In so doing, we see the traces of what has been called "audit culture" wherein data, targets, and indicators have become key in monitoring success and disciplining failure (Shore, 2008; Shore & Wright, 1999). In addition to arguing that the 90–90–90 targets offer a transparent discourse of accountability, the 90–90–90 targets also produce, we argue, a way of making the HIV pandemic commensurable across space. They have provided a universal set of targets that are seemingly neutral and able to track progress towards the end of AIDS.

However, the perceived universality of numerical metrics such as the 90–90–90 targets is also important as a rhetorical device that acts as numbers that can synchronize various actors in the global HIV/AIDS effort. Leclerc-Madlala et al. have, in the context of the introduction of the 90–90–90 targets within PEPFAR, commented that "the task of getting a vastly heterogeneous global AIDS community on-board for the project of ending AIDS required consensus building, not only to establish support for the 2030 vision but also to establish a common language for the project" (2018, p. 974). This common language, we argue, was the introduction of the 90–90–90 targets: numerical metrics that were perceived to be able to transcend the local epidemic variations and the heterogeneous cultural, economic, and political contexts that the HIV epidemic is embedded within. Paraphrasing Dalsgaard, who has commensurability concerning carbon, we can state that the 90–90–90 targets provide a set of universal metrics that seem to be able to "transform different qualities within the HIV epidemic into a common set of metrics" (2013). The differences within the global HIV epidemic are made commensurable through the 90–90–90 targets that allow for comparability across all scales. In this way, the 90–90–90 targets also act as a new standardized way of tracking progress towards the end of AIDS. Standardization is, of course, a key aspect of making the world commensurable, and, as Theodore Porter has noted, the process of standardization is often conducted through recourse to numerical metrics and statistics (1986, 1996). There is, of course, a broad range of standardization techniques within the HIV epidemic, including the standardization of HIV tests, treatment guidelines, epidemiological categorization, and other protocols and technologies. Yet, as Espeland and Stevens note, "what distinguishes commensuration from other forms of standardization is the common metric it provides" (1998, p. 316). We argue that the 90–90–90 targets provide the global HIV effort with precisely this form of commensuration through a common set of metrics. The common language becomes a way of making the many local HIV epidemics commensurable across space and differences, rendering these local differences comparable through a common set of metrics.

Reviewing the numbers: what about the 10–10–10?

The 90–90–90 targets seem ambitious and bold, both in what the numbers say and what the model stipulates. Yet the 90–90–90 targets are also filled with embedded shortcomings. The targets themselves indeed anticipate that within a step of the targets, there will be those that do not get tested, those that do not access treatment, and, finally, those that will not achieve viral load suppression. In addition to this, the numbers of people who will not reach the targets grow from one metric to the next. If we here use the denominator of *all people living with HIV*, then the 90–90–90 targets' anticipated shortcomings translate to 90–81–73; thus, the targets themselves acknowledge implicitly that 10% won't get tested, 19% will not receive treatment, and 27% will not be virally suppressed.

Adams et al. have pointed to the function of anticipation in global health care and technoscience (2009), and the 90–90–90 targets seem to be an example of such a politics of anticipation. On the one hand, UNAIDS envisions that the path to an end to the HIV epidemic is through the 90–90–90 targets; however, at the same time, the very mathematical model of reaching the 90–90–90 targets anticipates and produces its outside. Alternatively, put in terms of synchronicity, it produces its non-synchronous outside with people who are anticipated to be left outside of the fulfillment of the 90–90–90 targets.

This begs the question, states Judith Auerbach: "who are the other 10–10–10, or rather, who are the other 10–19–27 who are not reached or engaged in the treatment cascade" (Auerbach, 2019, p. 100). It is outside the scope of this chapter to answer this question, but a summary is to provide a critique of the 90–90–90 targets both as the alleged guarantee towards the end of AIDS as well as noting the shortcomings of the model.

In brief, Auerbach points out that there are vast differences globally in terms of people knowing their status, but that in 2017, data showed that out of eighty-two countries representing 92% of the global HIV burden, only four had reached the first 90 target, and only eighteen had reached numbers between 70% and 89%

of people knowing their HIV status (Auerbach, 2019, p. 100). Similarly, global numbers from 2017 showed that in the second 90, accessing treatment, there were large gaps and differences across the globe. Numbers ranged from 85% on treatment in Western Europe and North America to 29% on treatment in the Middle East and North Africa (Auerbach, 2019, p. 101). Finally, the story is not much different within the last 90, people who are virally suppressed. Here, too, we find large global differences in how many achieve viral suppression. In the Middle East, for instance, only 22% of PLHIV were reported as having a suppressed viral load, while in North America and Western Europe, the numbers were as high as 65% (UNAIDS, 2018). Once again, the local differences here are stark. While North America has seen more and more people reaching viral suppression, disparities still exist, and data from San Francisco, for instance, show that young people and women, both cis and transgender, are less likely to achieve viral suppression than older adults and men (Garcia et al., 2017).

Finally, another problem with the 90–90–90 targets lies in their linear understanding or portrayal of "reaching" these goals. On the national level, this can mean that countries fall in and out of the list of countries that have reached these numbers, as numbers can fluctuate and are time bound. For people, this can mean that they are in and out of care, and this influences how viral suppression is maintained (Auerbach, 2019, p. 101). HIV treatment and care are not a linear process, either at the national level or the personal level of people living with HIV. The "end of AIDS," barring an effective vaccine or cure, is thus not an *event* but a continual process that needs to be understood as such.

Critique of the politics of counting

An additional critique of the 90–90–90 targets is that they firmly focus on treatment. While treatment is key and crucial to the overall success of HIV efforts, several scholars and community activists and affected community members have drawn attention to the need for *other* indicators and targets that go beyond the treatment paradigm. Some have drawn attention to the need for a "fourth 90," which often is conceptualized through the framework of quality of life (Harris et al., 2018; Lazarus et al., 2016). As Auerbach states, good health and quality of life are not part of the 90–90–90 targets, and data on this amongst people living with HIV is not collected as part of the official UNAIDS framework; thus, it is not measured (2019, p. 101). Since viral load suppression, for most people living with HIV, is not the end-all, be-all, it is important to consider that it is possible that, for some people living with HIV, quality of life might involve discontinuation of ARV if they tire of it or if it is a reminder of living where chronic adherence is expected to continue throughout their lives (Auerbach, 2019, p. 101). In offering this critique, we can start to see the many tensions that have come to occupy global health efforts related to HIV but also how metrics and indicators have come to take center stage on the road towards the end of AIDS. It also should remind us that these aspects of the HIV epidemic are not only political or even technical in nature. They are highly lived and social phenomena. Finally, the usage and reliance on the

90–90–90 targets also highlight how the world of HIV is made commensurable through metrics that at times obfuscate as much as they illuminate.

Another key critique of the "politics of counting" comes from the work of Sara Davis' notion of "the politics of the *uncounted*" (Davis, 2017, 2020; Davis et al., 2017). Davis' work points to how the governing HIV efforts through the usage of metrics as guides can obfuscate as much as they purport to illuminate. A case in point from Davis' work would be how so-called "key population estimates" are used in establishing a baseline metric for counting "key population size" within countries. In brief, the calculation of key populations is based on statistical calculations based on national and international surveys as well as demographic data. Through calculation, nations provide an estimate of the "prevalence" of how many men who have sex with men or transgender women there are within a given population, and based on this baseline, one can calculate, for instance, the percent of men who have sex with men who have tested for HIV. However, as Davis' work shows, many nations, in particular nations that have punitive laws against sex between men, underreport the size of the population that would be categorized as men who have sex with men (Davis, 2017; Davis et al., 2017). This problem is even more visible in categorizing transgender women, for instance. Thus, the politics of counting as envisioned by the 90–90–90 targets should be interrogated just as much by the politics of the *uncounted*. Rendered invisible in the data, this means that entire communities are being left behind and outside of the synchronized efforts to end AIDS. The metrics themselves produce communities of people who then become *outside of synchronization*.

Problematizing the role of indicators and metrics such as the 90–90–90 targets also involves an apparent anticipated result of the 90–90–90 targets. While the 90–90–90 targets were never intended to "end AIDS" per se, only to achieve "epidemic control," they still provide an important vista into how these targets also produce their outside, their non-synchronous subjects.

Our main concern, though, is to highlight how the establishment of the 90–90–90 targets and its subsequent counting can be seen as one of the tools or practices of synchronizing the end-of-AIDS narrative. The work of synchronization that the 90–90–90 targets do also includes the introduction of a framework for comparison; that is, since the 90–90–90 targets bring with them a universal language and a universal horizon of time, it allows for comparison between and across various geographical units. These units are either continental, regional, national, or even local and city level units of comparison (UNAIDS, 2017, 2018). In light of this comparative optic, temporality is also introduced through temporal linguistic markers such as "lagging," "keeping the pace," and "being off track" but also through charts and diagrams which introduce diagrammatic thinking around progress and the nature of tracking the end of AIDS.

Concluding remarks

This chapter seeks to explore how the 90–90–90 targets as a method and model for reaching the SDG target of "ending AIDS" within 2030 contain within themselves several potential pitfalls. These potential pitfalls are both linked to some of the normative effects that follow in the wake of the targets but also some of the more central debates around what sustainability is and how the very nature of sustainability becomes entangled with discourses of cost-effectiveness as well as the quantification of targets and goals.

We have tried to provide an abridged history of the end of AIDS as it has emerged in the wake of the 90–90–90 targets. In doing so, we have also tried to tease out how the 90–90–90 targets came to be, as well as how these targets, numerical as they are, also provide a narrative, a common language for diverse actors to rally around. One of the key points has been to highlight how, in the wake of an indicator-driven, data-dependent end to AIDS, as well as fiscal austerity, there has emerged a renewed focus on specific people and places. Sustainability through the discourse of numerical figures has meant a turn towards accountability, but accountability in the sense of making sure that one can account for the numbers and less the people. This seems to be at odds with the intended notion of sustainability when it comes to sexual health and, in this case, HIV prevention and treatment. In the previous, we have mapped some potential pitfalls of the ways in which sustainability, metrics, and accountability are entangled in the drive to "end AIDS." By providing this brief mapping, we hope to have opened up some critical reflections of the drive to end AIDS through the use of metrics and indicators while also looking at the more conceptual changes that have taken place within the usage of the concept of sustainability.

Notes

1 See the UNAIDS webpage on both resolutions. www.unaids.org/en/aboutunaids/unitednationsdeclarationsandgoals/unsecuritycouncilresolutions
2 See Res. 1308. www.unaids.org/sites/default/files/sub_landing/files/20000717_un_scresolution_1308_en.pdf
3 See Res.1983. www.unaids.org/sites/default/files/sub_landing/files/20110607_UNSC-Resolution1983_0.pdf
4 See the AVERT HIV timeline. www.avert.org/professionals/history-hiv-aids/overview
5 See the article presented in *New Scientist*. www.newscientist.com/article/dn4416-2003-worst-ever-year-for-hiv-says-un-report/
6 Ibid.
7 Ibid.
8 See the speech in full. www.unaids.org/en/speeches/2014/20141025_SP_EXD_Vietnam_launch_of_909090_en.pdf
9 See the recent PEPFAR strategies. www.state.gov/reports-pepfar/
10 See Devex. www.devex.com/news/what-s-behind-pepfar-s-funding-cut-threats-95053
11 Ibid.
12 Ibid.
13 See the article here: www.businesslive.co.za/bd/national/health/2019-04-10-health-department-scrambles-to-stop-us-cut-in-hiv-funds/
14 See Devex for more. www.devex.com/news/what-s-behind-pepfar-s-funding-cut-threats-95053
15 Ibid.
16 See Health Gap.org's report online. https://healthgap.org/pepfar-funding-cuts-threaten-the-future-of-people-living-with-hiv-in-kenya/

17 See Devex. www.devex.com/news/a-look-at-pepfar-s-strategy-controversies-and-motivations-93038
18 See the UNAIDS webpage. www.unaids.org/en/topic/data

References

Adams, V., Murphy, M., & Clarke, A. E. (2009). Anticipation: Technoscience, life, affect, temporality. *Subjectivity*, *28*(1), 246–265.
Adams, V., Novotny, T. E., & Leslie, H. (2008). Global health diplomacy. *Medical Anthropology*, *27*(4), 315–323.
Auerbach, J. D. (2019). Getting to zero begins with getting to ten. *Journal of Acquired Immune Deficiency Syndromes (1999)*, *82*(2), S99.
Center for Policy Impact in Global Health. (2019). *Health aid in transition a review of the U.S. President's Emergency Plan for Aids Relief (PEPFAR)*. http://centerforpolicyimpact.org/wp-content/uploads/sites/18/2019/09/PEPFAR-AID-Transition-Profile.pdf
Dalsgaard, S. (2013). The commensurability of carbon: Making value and money of climate change. *HAU: Journal of Ethnographic Theory*, *3*(1), 80–98.
Davis, S. L. (2017). The uncounted: Politics of data and visibility in global health. *The International Journal of Human Rights*, *21*(8), 1144–1163.
Davis, S. L. (2020). *The uncounted: Politics of data in global health*. Cambridge University Press.
Davis, S. L., Goedel, W. C., Emerson, J., & Guven, B. S. (2017). Punitive laws, key population size estimates, and global AIDS response progress reports: An ecological study of 154 countries. *Journal of the International AIDS Society*, *20*(1), 21386.
Engebretsen, E., Heggen, K., Das, S., Farmer, P., & Ottersen, O. P. (2016). Paradoxes of sustainability with consequences for health. *The Lancet Global Health*, *4*(4), e225–e226.
Espeland, W. N., & Stevens, M. L. (1998). Commensuration as a social process. *Annual Review of Sociology*, *24*(1), 313–343.
Feldman, I., & Ticktin, M. (2010). *In the name of humanity: The government of threat and care*. Duke University Press.
Garcia, B., Aragon, T., & Scheer, S. (2017). *HIV epidemiology annual report 2016*. Department of Public Health Population Health Division.
Harris, T. G., Rabkin, M., & El-Sadr, W. M. (2018). Achieving the fourth 90: Healthy aging for people living with HIV. *AIDS (London, England)*, *32*(12), 1563.
Kenworthy, N. J. (2014). Global health: The debts of gratitude. *Women's Studies Quarterly*, *42*(1–2), 69–85.
Kenworthy, N. J., & Parker, R. (2014). *HIV scale-up and the politics of global health*. Taylor & Francis.
Kenworthy, N. J., Thomann, M., & Parker, R. (2018). Critical perspectives on the "end of AIDS". *Global Public Health*, 1–3.
Lachenal, G. (2013). A genealogy of treatment as prevention (TASP): Prevention, therapy, and the tensions of public health in African history. *Global Health in Africa: Historical Perspectives on Disease Control*, 70–91.
Lazarus, J. V., Safreed-Harmon, K., Barton, S. E., Costagliola, D., Dedes, N., del Amo Valero, J., Gatell, J. M., Baptista-Leite, R., Mendão, L., Porter, K., Vella, S., & Rockstroh, J. K. (2016). Beyond viral suppression of HIV – the new quality of life frontier. *BMC Medicine*, *14*(1), 94.
Leclerc-Madlala, S., Broomhall, L., & Fieno, J. (2018). The "end of AIDS" project: Mobilising evidence, bureaucracy, and big data for a final biomedical triumph over AIDS. *Global Public Health*, *13*(8), 972–981.

Lo, S., & Horton, R. (2015). AIDS and global health: The path to sustainable development. *The Lancet, 386*(9989), 106–108. https://doi.org/10.1016/S0140-6736(15)61040-6

PEPFAR. (2017). *Building a sustainable future: Report on the 2016 PEPFAR sustainability indices and dashboards (SIDs)*. https://www.state.gov/wp-content/uploads/2019/08/Building-a-Sustainable-Future-Report-on-the-2016-PEPFAR-Sustainability-Indices-and-Dashboards-SIDs.pdf

Piot, P. (2003). *AIDS: The need for an exceptional response to an unprecedented crisis.* UNAIDS Presidential Fellows Lecture, UNAIDS.

Porter, T. M. (1986). *The rise of statistical thinking, 1820–1900.* Princeton University Press.

Porter, T. M. (1996). *Trust in numbers: The pursuit of objectivity in science and public life.* Princeton University Press.

Resolution. (2015). *Transforming our world: The 2030 agenda for sustainable development.* Resolution adopted by the General Assembly on 25: 70/1. Seventieth United Nations General Assembly.

Rhodes, T., & Lancaster, K. (2020). Mathematical models as public troubles in COVID-19 infection control: Following the numbers. *Health Sociology Review*, 1–18.

Rhodes, T., Lancaster, K., & Rosengarten, M. (2020). A model society: Maths, models and expertise in viral outbreaks. *Critical Public Health*, 1–4. https://doi.org/10.1080/09581596.2020.1748310

Shore, C. (2008). Audit culture and illiberal governance: Universities and the politics of accountability. *Anthropological Theory, 8*(3), 278–298.

Shore, C., & Wright, S. (1999). Audit culture and anthropology: Neo-liberalism in British higher education. *Journal of the Royal Anthropological Institute*, 557–575.

Sibanda, A. (2000). A nation in pain: Why the HIV/AIDS epidemic is out of control in Zimbabwe. *International Journal of Health Services, 30*(4), 717–738.

UNAIDS. (2014). *90-90-90: An ambitious treatment target to help end the AIDS epidemic.* www.unaids.org/sites/default/files/media_asset/90-90-90_en.pdf

UNAIDS. (2017). *Ending AIDS: Progress towards the 90-90-90 targets. Global AIDS update.* UNAIDS.

UNAIDS. (2018). *Miles to go – closing gaps, breaking barriers, righting injustices.* Document 268. UNAIDS.

7 Conclusion

Sustainable sexual health as governmentality?

Introduction

Sustainability and sexual health: two buzzwords within the current paradigm of global and public health. While initially, it might not be self evident that these two terms are entangled, we have tried to show that even from the outset of Malthusian concerns with "sustainable yields," overpopulation, and the "onto-logical trap," there was always a relationship between the two concepts. Even though this relationship was not fully articulated nor framed within any official paradigm as we now see it with the SDGs, sexuality was part and parcel of this genealogy. In the SDG era, we more and more see a fully articulated connec-tion being drawn between these two terms: in policy documents, strategies, and reports. In this concluding chapter, we want to reflect a bit on what we have teased out in the past chapters, but more so, we also want to offer some glimpses into a (speculative) future and what it can mean and will mean to have sustain-able sexual health.

We have, in this book, mapped several different yet entangled cases where sexual health has been at the foreground while sustainability has been in the background, emerging from time to time. The many sources we have ana-lyzed have mainly been textual, and as such, we have also tried to highlight the importance of "prescriptive" documents. Of course, a word of caution is in order here: while we have tried, at least implicitly, to highlight the pro-ductiveness of texts, we acknowledge that the texts themselves have a rather problematic analytical value attached to them. First of all, the documents we have analyzed mask the often troubled and conflict-filled space in which they are made. A case in point would be the SDGs themselves: the SDGs and the Agenda 2030 document, when read standing alone, give the impression that the SDGs themselves were made in a consensus-filled manner. Yet, the SDGs themselves and the many targets and goals were the objects of conflicts, nego-tiations, and pragmatic compromises. As Steven Epstein stated in a slightly different setting (1996, p. 355), our goal has been to analytically juxtapose contemporary records and sources in an effort to highlight how "different social worlds" comment upon, and make sense of, various strategies towards sustain-able sexual health. Our analytical cue has been to assume that different social worlds and different actors and stakeholders engage differently in the construction of a narrative that subscribes to the notion that sexual health matters and is made to matter in the SDG era. Bringing an eclectic set of sources and themes into proximity, as we have done in this book, allows us, we argue, to analyze how different stakeholders, actors, and mediums construct, relate to, and configure sexual health and sustainability.

There is, of course, a caveat here which pertains to the previous insights: published stories only tell part of this story, as Epstein noted in his work (1996, p. 355). The same is true for our story in this book. In using textual sources, we must also remember that these represent the end result of an oftentimes long and even contested process of becoming finished texts. "Sometimes, in their linearity and smoothness, finished documents *conceal* the story" (Epstein, 1996, p. 355, original italics). Indeed, this is a pitfall of our analysis; textual sources, even when they come from different sources and domains, can only provide us with an overarching thematic structure of how sexual health has come to matter. Yet the claims made should be taken as part of a *narrative analysis* of sexual health and sustainability discourses, one that seeks to problematize *why, how, and what effects* sexual health strategies, reports, and goals produce under the umbrella of sustainability.

Part of this book's rationale has been to uncover some of the tensions and paradoxes that have emerged in the age of the SDGs and the subsequent effects when they are acted out in strategies and plans for sexual health. In so doing, we have also tried to map the relationship between the individual, the nation, and the global: between scales and actors. In this last part of this concluding chapter, we will dedicate some space to two topics which are related: what it means to govern in the name of sustainability and the future of sustainability and its repercussions for sexual health.

Governing in the name of sustainability

We have argued throughout this book that sustainability has become a buzzword within global health governance and beyond. Sustainability has taken hold even within the domain of sexual and reproductive health and rights discourses. As such, sustainability has become what Foucault might have called "a governmental strategy" (2007). For Foucault, a governmental strategy, also called "governmentality," can be understood as the organized practices through which subjects are governed (Mayhew, 2015). The very term "governmentality" is often understood to also signify problems of self-control, guidance for the family and for children, management of the household, and the directing of the soul (Lemke, 2001, p. 191). However, in recent scholarship, the term "governmentality" has taken on a broad semantic meaning and has come to include definitions such as "the art of government" (Burchell et al., 1991), "the techniques and strategies by which a society is rendered governable" (Lemke, 2002), or, most famously, "the conduct of conduct" (Foucault, 2007). Thomas Lemke has stated that "Foucault defines government as conduct, or, more precisely, as 'the conduct of conduct' and thus as a term that ranges from 'governing the self' to 'governing others'" (2002, p. 51). In short, governmentality

> plays a decisive role in his analytics of power in several regards: it offers a view on power beyond a perspective that centers either on consensus or on violence; it links technologies of the self with technologies of domination, the constitution of the subject to the formation of the state; and finally, it helps to differentiate between power and domination.
>
> (Lemke, 2002, p. 52)

So what does it mean when we now, at the end of this book, claim that sustainability has become a governmental strategy?

In this book, we have argued that sexual health strategies in the era of the SDGs have at times both explicit and implicit connections to sustainability thinking. To govern sexual health in today's climate is predicated upon a vast range of technologies, mentalities, and measures, yet many of these are rolled out and scaled up in the name of sustainability. The "end of AIDS" is one such example, as are PEPFAR's HIV strategies. Sexual health reports and strategies, as we have seen, also mix in the language of sustainability as a way of framing and grounding sexual health governance. As such, sustainability has become more and more a way of governing subjects and in turn sexual health.

However, what does it mean to govern in a sustainable fashion? When all 193 member states of the UN ratified and signed the 2030 Agenda document, and all the heads of states of the member states proclaimed that

> We are resolved to free the human race from the tyranny of poverty and want and to heal and secure our planet. We are determined to take the bold and transformative steps which are urgently needed to shift the world onto a sustainable and resilient path. As we embark on this collective journey, we pledge that no one will be left behind.
>
> (Resolution, 2015, p. 1)

who is actually speaking here? Moreover, what does this have to say for sexual health governance? By way of a small detour, we shall in the following lay out some of the ways in which sustainability discourse might be read as more and more a governmental practice or, more aptly, a way of influencing the "conduct of conduct."

A key phrase in the current discourse on sustainability and the SDGs has been the goal that the SDGs will seek to improve the conditions of all of humanity and thus "leave no one behind" on the road to a better world in 2030. This has, of course, also come to influence sexual health thinking, as we have seen in the WHO European region's strategic plan for sexual health as well as UNAIDS' framework for ending AIDS and, finally, PEPFAR's work on the HIV pandemic. Yet what does it mean to "leave no one behind"? Who is ensuring that "we" will not leave anyone behind? Moreover, who is at risk of being left behind?

By proclaiming that "no one will be left behind," a universal promise seems to be made on behalf of humanity and, at the same time, to humanity by a universal humanity. Such governance in the name of a common humanity has been seen before and analyzed in an anthology edited by Ilana Feldman and Miriam Ticktin titled *In the Name of Humanity: The Government of Threat and Care* (2010). Here Feldman and Ticktin describe the paradox of governing in and through recourse to the concept of "humanity." Humanity can act as a unifying concept for humanitarian interventions (Feldman & Ticktin, 2010, pp. 238–256), global medical aid (Feldman & Ticktin, 2010, pp. 151–190), and ecological initiatives in preserving ecological systems (Feldman & Ticktin, 2010, pp. 190–238). However, as Feldman and Ticktin also show, to govern or to intervene in the name of humanity also implies engaging in military operations, such as the case in Iraq (2010, pp. 1–27) or the Balkans. It might also be used in a biomedical setting to test out new drug candidates outside of the Global North by "offshoring" clinical trials (Feldman & Ticktin, 2010, pp. 218–238). Finally, it might also mean invoking the rhetoric of humanity when governments engage in "the war on terror" and implement various surveillance programs and legal mechanisms to "combat terror in the name of humanity" (Reid, 2013). Other examples outside of Feldman and Ticktin can be taken from various pandemic or epidemics; here the Ebola epidemic and the militarization of medical aid that followed in the wake of the 2014 Ebola epidemic are good examples of resorting to governance in the name of humanity (Benton, 2014; Burci, 2014; Park & Umlauf, 2014). Another example can be seen in the response to the "bird flu" or the H1N1 pandemic, which also gives credence to the various ways in which the rhetoric of governing in the name of humanity is utilized (Caballero-Anthony, 2006; Stephenson, 2011). Finally, the ongoing COVID-19 pandemic has triggered a global response never seen before in modern history: here, vast lockdowns across the globe with subsequent travel bans and social distancing measures have all been conducted in the name of humanity in order to control the pandemic.

Governing in the name of humanity and sustainability has several overlapping commonalities but also some differences which we want to surface here at the end of our analysis of sexual health and sustainability.

Much like the issue of governing in the name of humanity, so too does the recourse to governing in the name of sustainability presuppose a broad range of political and ethical imaginaries (Feldman & Ticktin, 2010, p. 3). Moreover, like the use of the trope of acting in the name of humanity, so too does the invoking of governing and acting in the name of sustainability have demonstrable and significant effects upon the lives of people, effects that also show us that to govern in the name of sustainability is also ever and always a normative exercise of power. It is almost uncanny how acting on behalf of humanity, on the one hand, and, on the other hand, how to govern in the name of a sustainable future invoke many of the same tropes and rhetorical statements. Perhaps this is because humanity's future depends on a shift that will change the current pace of things and thus transform humanity's common future into a sustainable one. Or perhaps it is because the sustainable development goals frame the drive for a sustainable future with recourse to a universal category of humanity. The recourse to a common and universal category of humanity, or a universal "we," can be deconstructed, and through this deconstructive reading, as we have shown earlier, what on the surface of it might seem like a universalist category quickly breaks down, and the burden of ensuring a sustainable future is shifted onto several more localized "we" actors. The question of governing in the name of sustainability is, just like that of governing in the name of humanity, built on, as stated, ethical and political considerations. It is also built on certain epistemological rationales as well as creating binaries upon which sustainability can be made to act in such a way as to *make something sustainable*.

In UN Resolution A/70/L.1, or the Agenda 2030 resolution, it is stated that

> On behalf of the peoples we serve, we have adopted a historic decision on a comprehensive, far-reaching and people-centered set of universal and trans-formative Goals and targets . . . as we embark on this great collective journey, we pledge that no one will be left behind. Recognizing that the dignity of the human person is fundamental, we wish to see the Goals and targets met for all nations and peoples and for all segments of society. And we will endeavor to reach the furthest behind first.
>
> (Resolution, 2015, p. 3)

In this excerpt, we see that there is a universal sense of *the human* as well as a notion of a *collective journey*, one that will leave *no one behind*. In short, sustainable development *is* universal and collective and is done for the betterment of all humans, that is, for all of humanity. However, thinking along these lines would not have been possible without what Thomas Laqueur has described as the emergence of humanity as a "sentiment" in the late 18th century (1989, 2009), a process which merges the concepts of "the human" with that of "the humane." In this process, humanity becomes a concept in which humans come to view themselves as ethical subjects in a humanitarian narrative; that is, by merging the human (wo/man as biological being) with that of the humane (an ethical disposition towards others), Laqueur suggests that this produced a narrative of obligation to treat one's fellow humans as connected, as being part of something larger than oneself (2003, p. 38). This is, of course, also covered in the idea of sustainable development, except here the ethical and political imperatives are no longer only aimed at being humane towards fellow humans but indeed have also come to mean that humans need to become humane towards the very ecosystem that has sustained us throughout history. In short, governing in the name of sustainability also means becoming humane towards nature.

There is also another way in which to govern in the name of humanity, or to intervene in the name of humanity, is similar or connected to that of a governmentality of sustainability. Humanity is frequently "defined by its breach," states Teitel (2004). Examples of these breaches which invoke the concept of humanity are the idea of the *inhumane*, such as war crimes, epidemics which cause great suffering and infirmity, and, finally, natural disasters and the subsequent disaster aid being mustered in the name of humanitarian help. As Feldman and Ticktin state so poignantly, in certain moments, the idea of invoking the concept of humanity as a governing mechanism is often less about making a claim about global connections than it is about the identification of universal threats (2010, p. 5).

So, too, is it when invoking sustainability as a mechanism for governing people through ethical and political injunctions. The UN Agenda once again can serve to illuminate this when the Resolution clearly defines the universal threats of today, which this rather long quote from the Resolution will show us:

> We are meeting at a time of immense challenges to sustainable development. Billions of our citizens continue to live in poverty and are denied a life of dignity. There are rising inequalities within and among countries. There are enormous disparities of opportunity, wealth, and power. Gender inequality remains a key challenge. Unemployment, particularly youth unemployment, is a major concern. Global health threats, more frequent and intense natural disasters, spiraling conflict, violent extremism, terrorism and related humanitarian crises and forced displacement of people threaten to reverse much of the development progress made in recent decades. Natural resource depletion and adverse impacts of environmental degradation, including desertification, drought, land degradation, freshwater scarcity and loss of biodiversity, add to and exacerbate the list of challenges that humanity faces. Climate change is one of the greatest challenges of our time and its adverse impacts undermine the ability of all countries to achieve sustainable development. Increases in global temperature, sea-level rise, ocean acidification and other climate change impacts are seriously affecting coastal areas and low-lying coastal countries, including many least developed countries and small island developing States. The survival of many societies, and of the biological support systems of the planet, is at risk.
>
> (Resolution, 2015, p. 5)

Besieged on all fronts, the UN's SDG Agenda resolution paints a picture wherein *humanity* is surrounded by existential risks, some the result of *inhumane* humans (such as terrorists and extremists) or *inhumane actions* such as "all forms of violence against all women and girls in the public and private spheres, including trafficking and sexual and other types of exploitation," as envisioned by SDG 5.2 (Resolution, 2015, p. 18), or all forms of "abuse, exploitation, trafficking and all forms of violence against and torture of children" specified by SDG 16.2 (Resolution, 2015, p. 25). Other threats are caused by climate change, once again caused by human activity but which nevertheless can be mitigated and combated by recourse to a common humanity which acts in *sustainable ways*. In the quote, both a governing through humanity and through sustainability are invoked. However, humanity and, in turn, sustainability only come to the fore through the breaches or universal threats, as both Teitel and Feldman and Ticktin point out. One of the common paradoxes shared by both the recourse to action in the name of humanity on the one hand and to sustainability on the other is that the threat to humanity and to a sustainable planet/humanity is most often other human beings (Feldman & Ticktin,

2010, p. 5). Sustainability as it is invoked by the UN is linked to sentiments that play on sympathy, compassion, and a universal human collective, the human race and humanity. Yet the very need for sustainable development and the various goals that come with it in the Agenda plan are also motivated by fear and insecurity for what the future might hold for *humanity*.

As such, this short exposé of the various commonalities between the concept of governing in the name of humanity and then governing in the name of sustainability has shown us that the two concepts are entangled in ways that produce both ethical sentiments and moral debates, as well as motivating political action. We have already taken this up earlier in the book by analyzing the preamble and the main content of the Agenda 2030 document in relation to what we have called the "double voicing paradox" of the implementation of the UN SDGs. We have done this to highlight two interrelated issues which have been of importance as this book has progressed; the first issue was to show how the Agenda document produces not a universal "we" but rather several smaller "we" actors who are then obligated to follow up on the SDGs and the "end of AIDS."

In the case of the universal "we" versus a smaller, plural "we," this becomes problematic, we have argued, as it creates obligations towards the smaller and plural "we," while the promise to end AIDS or to eradicate poverty is made in the name of a universal "we." To invoke a universal "we" that promises to ensure a sustainable future and, in this case, also the "end of AIDS," is at the same time an exercise in power, for it binds nations to make good on a universal promise while at the same time also leaving them, at times, to fend for themselves. Ultimately, we have shown that to govern in the name of sustainable sexual health binds individual subjects to the promise of ending AIDS, for instance; thus, what was, in the beginning, a collective and universal "we" becomes further down in the implementation chain and the intertextual network, a singularized obligation to end AIDS and to ensure sustainable maternal health.

Governing in the name of sustainability in an era when sexual health has become more and more visible both in policies and in global health has, as we have argued, meant the creation of tension-filled spaces. On the one hand, sustainability is framed as a promise in sexual health care discourses, yet it is often left up to local authorities and, in most cases, the individual subjects themselves to ensure that their sexual health is "sustainable." Sexual health in the era of the SDGs has also meant a greater drive towards quantification, big data, and biopharmaceuticals. Technology is seen as integral to the achievement of good national, communal, and personal sexual health. The same is true of the incorporation of a rights perspective and a pedagogy of sexual health and rights.

These are all laudable efforts and indeed also important in bringing more focus onto these topics, yet, as we also have seen, this has led to some paradoxes and tensions which might undermine the holistic ideology of sexual health as it has emerged through the years. Of particular note is the absence of any discourse around human pleasure as part of sexual health. We have also noted how, within the international HIV effort and the drive towards greater and greater quantification and indicator-driven interventions, there is an inherent risk that this might be counterproductive or at least risk leaving vulnerable people behind on the road to ending AIDS. We have dedicated space to both a historical trajectory of sustainability and the concept of sexual health while also offering a few case studies on different aspects of sexual health policies in the era of the SDGs. This has been both an exercise in retrospection but also in mapping contemporary issues. We now want to dedicate the last section of this concluding chapter to offering some perspectives for the future and what the future might hold for sexual health in the era of the SDGs.

Towards a sustainable future – leaving no one behind

Governing sexual health in the name of sustainability has meant to a large degree focusing on targets, indicators, and goals. It has meant creating strategies and reports which cover a broad range of topics yet also occlude some areas, such as pleasure. Finally, sexual health is still, albeit less so, also a normative concept. Its meaning has come to encompass a broad range of topics and issues and as such has come to be a highly polysemous term. So what can the future hold for such a concept and its connection with sustainability rhetoric? While we do not profess to offer a telling of the future, we can map some of the implications that the blind spots, tensions, and paradoxes that we have surfaced in this book can come to have.

In analyzing several European strategy plans for sexual health, as we did in Chapter 5, we clearly saw an omission of pleasure as part of sexual health. Indeed, the very term "pleasure" was clearly not included in these strategies. We argued, alongside Mamo and Epstein, that sexual health has become a buzzword and also a concept with highly polyvocal meaning content, which has meant that it can be used to address several different social issues. However, while Mamo and Epstein, in their original and well-argued study, arrive at this conclusion, we also contend that while sexual health can and does cover a broad range of issues, it nevertheless omits pleasure as part of its field of impact in official strategies.

If the SDGs and sustainability in general are predicated upon an idea of holistic and human-centered discourses, then the omission of pleasure as part of human sexual health seems counterintuitive to this. Sustainable sexual health should account for human pleasure and desire, as these are fundamental attributes of sexuality and thus also of health. We have come a long way in many ways when it comes to talking about and framing sexual health and sexual rights, yet pleasure seems still somewhat on the margins of sexual health. It should give us pause, then, that one of the core driving forces of human sexuality is all but forgotten in official strategies and reports. Even in those sections that deal with sexual health in pedagogy and in school curricula, pleasure is omitted. Instead, as we have seen, sexual health has a strong focus on biomedical aspects of health and sexuality: reducing STIs and HIV, reproductive health, and sexual function. A strong rights-based framework is also present, as is a strong emphasis on many of the strategies for boundary setting and learning about sexual and corporal autonomy. Yet learning about the role of pleasure and of love and desire is all but gone. The same goes for aspects of learning about the pleasurable aspects of sexuality as part of a healthy discourse of sex as mental and physical well-being. Indeed, one might ask how one can call any strategy sustainable which does not recognize the fundamental aspect of pleasure as part of sexual health. We can then, of course, ask a final question: How sustainable is it not to include pleasure as part of the official discourse of sexual health when pleasure is so fundamental to human sexuality and thus also human sexual health? The future might then be a future where this is also included, where Foucault's *ars erotica* is finally reunited with the current *scientia sexualis* and what emerges in the era of the SDGs is a truly holistic conceptualization of sexual health.

This brings us to another main point in this book, which has been the increasing quantification of human health, including sexual health, in the era of the SDGs and sustainability thinking.

All of the strategies and reports that we have analyzed in this book start out with aspirational goal setting and then a long list of targets to be reached and indicators to monitor progress towards these targets and their aspirational goals. The reliance on metrics and indicators in the era of the SDGs clearly has resonance in global health writ large, as Vinncane Adams has argued. While we are not arguing against good monitoring of progress on health indicators, nor do we in general oppose the use of metrics, our argument is that metrics and indicators might obscure issues, thus risking leaving people behind. We have seen this in the case of the 90–90–90 targets, as well as in the case of PEPFAR and the use of metrics as a way of leveraging political power. The politics of counting, or what Sara Davis has called the politics of the uncounted, also means that the use of indicators and metrics in sexual health might end up excluding certain groups if they are not counted or recognized. It also means that a lot of power is given to those who set the targets and thus also make the indicators, which in turn might undermine local perspectives on sexual health and what matters to local actors rather than governmental authorities or international organizations.

The future in this case might be towards the governance of sexual health where targets and indicators are negotiated together with the people who live in local contexts. While this might mean that we lose some of our abilities to compare and commensurate results, we might gain local engagement and perspectives on matters that are important on the ground for affected communities. There is, of course, a fine balance between atomizing data to such a degree that it can only have validity in specific contexts and, on the other hand, using such broad strokes that local nuances vanish. However, a starting point might be what Sara Davis observes in the context of the global HIV effort: to engage with local stakeholders and work with them in order to come up with meaningful targets for local communities while also at the same time seeing if these can be extrapolated to other settings. A sustainable future for the governance of sexual health might include, first of all, defining sustainability as something more than proving the ability of self-improvement through metrics. Second, it might also include engaging more with local communities in the process of making targets and indicators and even goals. This would ground sexual health priorities in the local communities themselves while also distributing power and engagement through networks ranging from global organization to nation states and finally to the local actors themselves. Sexual health, as has been argued throughout this book, is a concept that encompasses both the global population as well as the individual subject. Thus, what is needed is a sustainable politics of life where life is also understood to include the act wherein life can be made, that is, the intimate moment of sex. However, since sex is far from only a means of reproduction, we should also be privy to the politics of pleasure as part of the politics of sustainability.

Ultimately, what we need is a sustainable politics of life. We maintain that "if we are to take the UNs Sustainable Development Goals (SDGs) seriously, health can no longer be reduced to a purely biomedical concept" (Sandset et al., 2020, p. 1). The same goes for sexual health: sexual health can no longer be relegated to the domain of biomedicine proper and needs to be reintegrated into an holistic, rights-based framework which, moreover, is also embedded in the everyday lives of people where pleasure is part of such discourses of health.

References

Benton, A. (2014). The epidemic will be militarized: Watching outbreak as the West African Ebola epidemic unfolds. *Cultural Anthropology, 15.*

Burchell, G., Gordon, C., & Miller, P. (1991). *The Foucault effect: Studies in governmentality.* University of Chicago Press.

Burci, G. L. (2014). Ebola, the security council and the securitization of public health. *Questions of International Law, 10,* 27–39.

Caballero-Anthony, M. (2006). Combating infectious diseases in East Asia: Securitization and global public goods for health and human security. *Journal of International Affairs,* 105–127.

Epstein, S. (1996). *Impure science: AIDS, activism, and the politics of knowledge* (vol. 7). University of California Press.

Feldman, I., & Ticktin, M. (2010). *In the name of humanity: The government of threat and care.* Duke University Press.

Foucault, M. (2007). *Security, territory, population: Lectures at the Collège de France, 1977–78.* Springer.

Laqueur, T. W. (1989). Bodies, details, and the humanitarian narrative. *The New Cultural History, 176.*

Laqueur, T. W. (2003). *Solitary sex: A cultural history of masturbation.* Zone Books.

Laqueur, T. W. (2009). Mourning, pity, and the work of narrative in the making of "humanity". *Humanitarianism and Suffering: The Mobilization of Empathy,* 31–57.

Lemke, T. (2001). "The birth of bio-politics": Michel Foucault's lecture at the Collège de France on neo-liberal governmentality. *Economy and Society, 30*(2), 190–207.

Lemke, T. (2002). Foucault, governmentality, and critique. *Rethinking Marxism, 14*(3), 49–64.

Mayhew, S. (2015). *A dictionary of geography.* Oxford University Press.

Park, S. J., & Umlauf, R. (2014). Caring as existential insecurity: Quarantine, care, and human insecurity in the Ebola crisis. *Somatosphere.* http://somatosphere.net/2014/11/caring-as-existential-insecurity.html

Reid, J. (2013). *The biopolitics of the war on terror: Life struggles, liberal modernity, and the defence of logistical societies*. Manchester University Press.

Resolution. (2015). *Transforming our world: The 2030 agenda for sustainable development*. Resolution adopted by the General Assembly on 25: 70/1. Seventieth United Nations General Assembly.

Sandset, T. J., Heggen, K., & Engebretsen, E. (2020). What we need is a sustainable politics of life. *The Lancet, 395*.

Stephenson, N. (2011). Emerging infectious disease/emerging forms of biological sovereignty. *Science, Technology, & Human Values, 36*(5), 616–637. www.jstor.org/stable/23064911

Teitel, R. (2004). For humanity. *Journal of Human Rights, 3*(2), 225–237.

Index

Page numbers followed by 'n' indicate a note on the corresponding page.

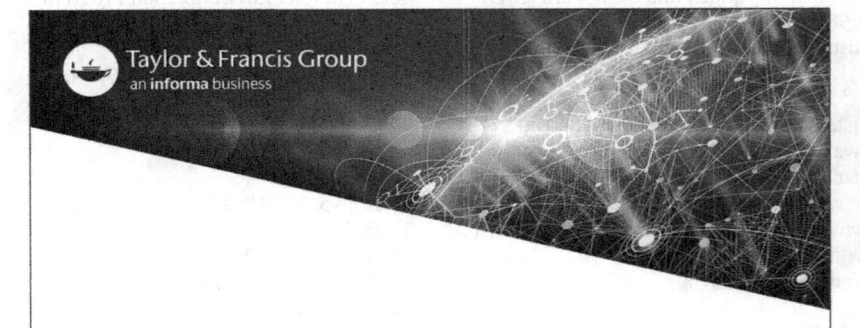
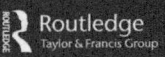
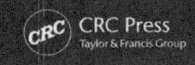